A Practical Guide to
Palliative Care

Jerry L. Old, MD

Chief Medical Officer
Hospice Care of Kansas/Voyager Hospice Care;
Clinical Assistant Professor of Family Medicine
University of Kansas School of Medicine
Kansas City, Kansas

Daniel L. Swagerty, Jr., MD, MPH

Associate Professor of Family Medicine and Internal Medicine
Director, Division of Geriatric Medicine and Palliative Care,
Department of Family Medicine
Associate Director, Landon Center on Aging
Director of Clinical Geriatrics,
University of Kansas School of Medicine
Kansas City, Kansas

. Wolters Kluwer | Lippincott Williams & Wilkins
Health

Philadelphia · Baltimore · New York · London
Buenos Aires · Hong Kong · Sydney · Tokyo

Acquisitions Editor: Sonya Seigafuse
Managing Editor: Nancy Winter
Production Manager: Bridgett Dougherty
Senior Manufacturing Manager: Benjamin Rivera
Marketing Manager: Kimberly Schonberger
Design Coordinator: Holly Reid McLaughlin
Cover Designer: Karen Quigley
Production Services: Nesbitt Graphics, Inc.
Printer: Quebecor World–Taunton

530 Walnut Street
Philadelphia, PA 19106 USA
LWW.com

Printed in the USA

Library of Congress Cataloging-in-Publication Data

A practical guide to palliative care / [edited by] Jerry L. Old, Daniel L. Swagerty.
  p. ; cm.
 Includes bibliographical references and index.
 ISBN 0-7817-6343-6
 1. Palliative treatment. 2. Hospice care. 3. Terminal care. I. Old, Jerry L.
II. Swagerty, Daniel.
 [DNLM: 1. Palliative Care. 2. Terminal Care. WB 310 P895 2007]
 R726.8.P695 2007
 616'.029—dc22

2007006975

Care has been taken to confirm the accuracy of the information presented and to describe
generally accepted practices. However, the authors, editors, and publisher are not responsible for errors or omissions or for any consequences from application of the information in
this book and make no warranty, expressed or implied, with respect to the currency, com-
pleteness, or accuracy of the contents of the publication. Application of this information in
a particular situation remains the professional responsibility of the practitioner.

The authors, editors, and publisher have exerted every effort to ensure that drug selection
and dosage set forth in this text are in accordance with current recommendations and practice at the time of publication. However, in view of ongoing research, changes in government regulations, and the constant flow of information relating to drug therapy and drug
reactions, the reader is urged to check the package insert for each drug for any change in
indications and dosage and for added warnings and precautions. This is particularly important when the recommended agent is a new or infrequently employed drug.

Some drugs and medical devices presented in this publication have Food and Drug Administration (FDA) clearance for limited use in restricted research settings. It is the responsibility of the health care provider to ascertain the FDA status of each drug or device planned
for use in their clinical practice.

To purchase additional copies of this book, call our customer service department at (800) 638
-3030 or fax orders to (301) 223-2320. International customers should call (301) 223-2300.

Visit Lippincott Williams & Wilkins on the Internet: at LWW.com. Lippincott Williams &
Wilkins customer service representatives are available from 8:30 am to 6 pm, EST.

10 9 8 7 6 5 4 3 2 1

A Practical Guide to

Palliative Care

This book is dedicated to Clara Lois Old and MaryAnn McMullan, our mothers, from whom we learned so much about life. After initial curative care interventions were unsuccessful for cancer diagnoses, they made the good decision to choose palliation over futile treatment. Death for them was a dignified, peaceful experience at home with family present as they passed to the hereafter. Neither of our families would have been able to care for them at home without the help and support of hospice, for which we are so very grateful.

Contents

SECTION 4 PREDICTING LIFE EXPECTANCY 87

Contents

SECTION 5 DELIVERY OF PALLIATIVE CARE 105

SECTION 6 TERMINAL CARE 119

SECTION 7 NONPAIN SYMPTOM MANAGEMENT 133

SECTION 8 PAIN CONTROL 175

EDITOR: Jerry L. Old

SECTION 9 PALLIATIVE INTERVENTIONS 235

EDITOR: Jerry L. Old

SECTION 10 THE PALLIATIVE PEDIATRIC PATIENT 259

EDITORS: Julia T. Raper, Ronald M. Perkin

SECTION 11 CHARTING 277

EDITOR: Jerry L. Old

SECTION 12 ETHICS AT THE END OF LIFE 293

EDITOR: Jerry L. Old

Contributors

Margaret L. Barnett, ARNP, BC-PCM
Palliative Care Clinical Nurse Specialist
Department of Nursing
University of Kansas Hospital
Kansas City, Kansas

Nellie Kay Dimmitt RN, MS
Director of Education
Hospice Care of Kansas and the Midwest,
  LLC
Lenexa, Kansas

Rick Hall, RN
Certified Wound Care Consultant
Hospice Care of Kansas
Wichita, Kansas;
Hospice Care of the Midwest
Kansas City, Missouri

Martha Johnson-Swagerty, RN
Executive Director
Hospice Care of America
Rockford, Illinois

Jerry L. Old, MD
Chief Medical Officer
Hospice Care of Kansas/Voyager Hospice Care
Clinical Assistant Professor of Family Medicine
University of Kansas School of Medicine
Kansas City, Kansas

Ronald M. Perkin, MD, MA
Professor and Chairman
Department of Pediatrics
Brody School of Medicine at East Carolina
  University;
Medical Director, Children's Hospital
University Health Systems of Eastern Carolina
Greenville, North Carolina

Karin Porter-Williamson, MD
Assistant Professor
Department of General and Geriatric Medicine
University of Kansas School of Medicine;
Attending Physician
Palliative Care Service
University of Kansas Hospital
Kansas City, Kansas

Julia T. Raper, RN, MSN
Administrator
Children's Hospital
University Health Systems of Eastern Carolina
Greenville, North Carolina

Daniel L. Swagerty Jr., MD, MPH
Associate Professor of Family Medicine and
  Internal Medicine
Director, Division of Geriatric Medicine and
  Palliative Care,
Department of Family Medicine
Associate Director, Landon Center on Aging;
Director of Clinical Geriatrics,
University of Kansas School of Medicine
Kansas City, Kansas

Introduction

Over the years we have made a lot of discoveries—one of which is that end-of-life care is very rewarding. One cannot say it is fun, but it certainly is rewarding. There is no other area of medicine where there is so much need and so much potential to touch a patient's very existence.

As with any new specialty, hospice and palliative medicine is not well understood by either the public or the medical profession. This is not a comfortable topic.

However, good end-of-life care is something that medicine must do. After all, we are often part of the problem. By curing many of the acute ailments, we have created chronic disease. The dying process has become more complex, and now takes much longer. People in this country now live an average of thirty months after they receive a terminal diagnosis. In addition to the human impact, there is also a huge economic impact. By some estimates, the average patient will spend 75% of the entire healthcare dollars they have spent during their entire lifetime, during those last thirty months.

We must treat suffering as well as disease. Sometimes in treating the disease, with modern technology, we become the source of the suffering itself. The wise healthcare provider knows when to transition from cure to palliation.

This book is intended to be simple, succinct, and practical for everyone who may take care of a patient near the end of life. Much of palliative care is just common sense. The book is not a dark, deep text about a somber topic—but we have attempted to present palliative care in a light, yet dignified manner. Hospice/palliative care is about LIFE! It's about giving our patients the highest quality of life, for as long as possible, even if cure is not possible. This is the most noble thing that medicine can do. Just as we strive to provide a good birth, we must also strive to provide a good exit from this world.

Jerry L. Old, MD
Daniel L. Swagerty Jr., MD, MPH

The Palliative Care Approach

CHAPTER 1

Definitions

There will **ALWAYS** come a time when there is **nothing more** you can do to cure your **patient's disease**, but there is **ALWAYS** something you can do for your patient.

The mortality rate is still very close to 100%.

PALLIATIVE CARE

The term *palliative care* comes from the Greek language and literally means to "cloak" or to surround your patient with caring. That doesn't sound like "giving up" or "no care," as many health professionals conceive of palliative care, does it? The term "comfort care," when broken down, is "com—forte," which means to "care with strength." It implies aggressive care to provide comfort. That is the basis of Hospice and Palliative Medicine.

Palliative care is:

- Treatment that focuses on relieving suffering and improving quality of life of seriously ill patients
- Can be offered at any stage of illness
- Is NOT "no care" and often means aggressive care, such as in pain and symptom management
- Interdisciplinary care
- Personal, psychological, social, and spiritual support
- Bereavement support
- The newest Boarded Specialty (organized in 1995; formally recognized 2006) American Academy of Hospice and Palliative Medicine (www.abhpm.org/)

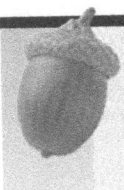

Definition of Palliative Care
IN A NUTSHELL

Palliative care is aggressive treatment of a patient's symptoms, when cure might not be possible, in order to provide the greatest quality of life, for as long as possible.

CHAPTER 2

Philosophy—from "Cure" to "Comfort"

Good end-of-life care is very **individual**, based upon the patient's philosophy of life, and their goals (1).

CONTRASTING VIEWS AT THE END OF LIFE

Not surprisingly, there are two opposing views of end-of-life treatment held by patients and health care workers:

I'm ready to go to Heaven!

- **The Emily Dickinson view—**

  "Ample make this bed,
  Make this bed with awe!
  In it wait 'til judgment break...
  Excellent and fair..."

  - These are the patients that usually have strong spiritual values and plan for a **peaceful death**.

  - Patients reach acceptance easily and may actually look forward to "going to Heaven!"

  - They seem to actually give those of us remaining strength.

I'm a fighter! Never Give Up!

- **The Dylan Thomas view—**

  "Do not go gentle into that good night...
  Rage! Rage!
  Against the dying of the light..."

  - This is the **"fighter!"**

- "Never give up!" (The traditional oncologist view!)
- "0.001% chance of cure—Sure! I want to try things that have been proven to not work too!"

OUR JOB

It's not that one or the other of the above philosophies on end-of-life is right or wrong. We cannot make that judgment. Our job is:

- To **"read" the patient's attitude/philosophy** and to be able to respond to it.
- We need a **reparatory of responses** to deal with both these types of patients, and all those in between.

> As health care professionals, we must NOT force our own end-of-life philosophy upon a vulnerable patient!

THE PATIENT'S GOALS

We must find out what the patient's **goals** are, and try to satisfy them (2). Once the patient's philosophy and **goals** are known, knowing how to care for that individual becomes much easier.

At some point, almost everyone begins to see his or her **goal as a good and peaceful death** (3).

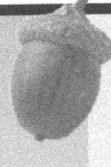

Philosophy—from "Cure" to "Comfort"
IN A NUTSHELL

Once a patient's philosophy about the end-of-life and their **goals** are determined, palliative care is much easier.

The **peaceful death**—"I'm ready for God to take me!"

The **fighter**—"I'm a fighter and will never give up—if I try hard enough I will beat this cancer!"

Our goal is to provide support, appropriate care, and quality of life to both types of patients, and all those in between.

The overall **mortality rate remains 100%.**

REFERENCES

1. Saunders C, ed. The Management of Terminal Disease. London: Edward Arnold Ltd.; 1978.
2. Storey P, Knight CF. UNIPAC One. *The Hospice/Palliative Medicine Approach to End-of-Life Care*. 2nd ed. Glenview, Illinois: American Academy of Hospice and Palliative Medicine; 2003.
3. Taylor GJ, Kurent JE. A Clinical Guide to Palliative Care. Blackwell Publishing; 2003.

CHAPTER **3**

The Transition from "Diagnose and Treat" to "Palliate"

Modern medicine is in the **"cure" mode**. Every symptom, every problem a patient has is seen as a challenge to **"diagnose and treat"** it. The only goal we often recognize is cure. With cure as the goal, we are assured of ultimately failing! The wise practitioner **does not "give up"** on his/her patient, but recognizes when it is time to **transition from "diagnose and treat" to "palliate"** (1). Figure 1 shows the **curative model** (2).

In the curative model, we **diagnose and treat** each problem that arises. Eventually death occurs ("we lost the patient"), and everyone is **shocked and surprised**.

Notice in the **palliative model** (Fig. 2) that supportive care and symptom control **start early**. As the terminal disease progresses, there is **less "diagnose and treat"** and **more "palliation."** Once the patient reaches hospice, treatment is all palliation. Then comes death—**no one is surprised** (patient, family, health care providers) because this has been evolving; and then everyone is **better prepared** for the bereavement that follows.

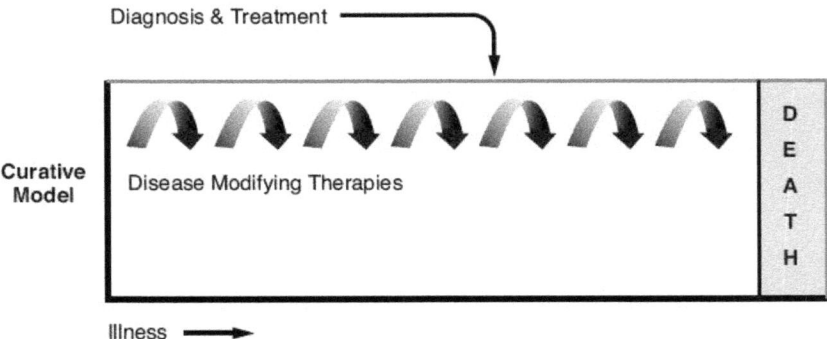

FIGURE 1 ● Curative model. (From World Health Organization: Cancer Pain Relief and Palliative Care. Technical Report Series 804. Geneva, Switzerland; 1990.)

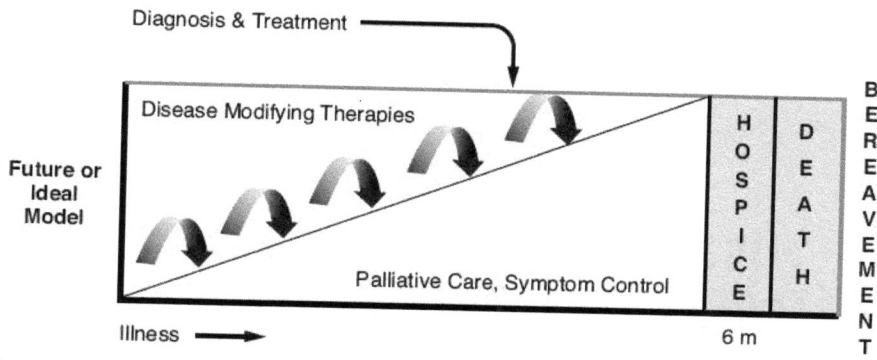

FIGURE 2 ● Palliative model.

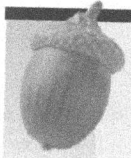

The Transition from "Diagnose and Treat" to "Palliate"
IN A NUTSHELL

Once a terminal diagnosis is established, a smooth transition from "diagnose and treat" to "palliation" is appropriate (3).

REFERENCES

1. Goodlin S. Framework for improving care. In: American Academy of Hospice and Palliative Medicine Bulletin. Available at: http://www.aahpm.org. Accessed August 20, 2006.
2. World Health Organization: Cancer Pain Relief and Palliative Care. Technical Report Series 804. Geneva, Switzerland; 1990.
3. Caring connections—What is hopice? Available at: http://www.caringinfo.org. Accessed August 15, 2006.

CHAPTER 4

Historical Perspective: What Has Changed?

The medical profession has created **Chronic Disease**! (1) In the past, life expectancy was low and death rates were high. The "Dying Trajectory" was short (2). That is, we were relatively healthy until we got sick—then we died, mostly from infectious diseases (Fig. 3). People did not live long enough to die from chronic diseases.

    Before the 20th century, very **few truly curable diseases** existed. Health professionals channeled their energies into **palliating and alleviating symptoms**.

> 18th century aphorism:
> To cure sometimes
> To relieve often
> To comfort always

    By the early to mid 20th century, vaccines, antibiotics, anesthetics, and improved diagnostic techniques and surgical procedures became reality. Suddenly the incurable became curable! Subtle changes took place in the psyche of health professionals as the **nature of medicine changed from palliation to cure**.

> 20th century aphorism:
> To comfort sometimes
> To relieve often
> To cure always

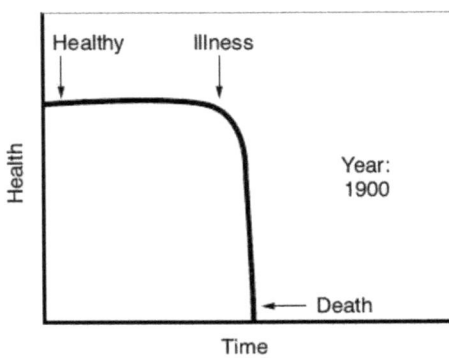

FIGURE 3 ⬤ Dying trajectory prior to the mid-1900s.

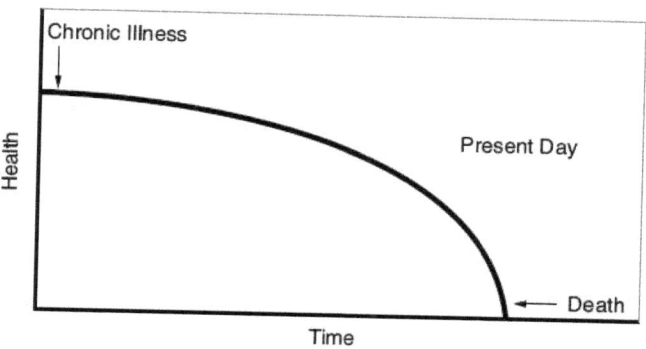

FIGURE 4 ● Dying has become more complex, taking an average of 30 months today.

Health care professionals began to accept **nothing short of cure**. As a result, **the era of chronic diseases** was born. The old dying trajectory changed. Dying has become more complex and takes much longer. People now live long enough to die from things like congestive heart failure, chronic obstructive pulmonary disease (COPD), cancers, renal failure, Alzheimer's disease (which may take 8–12 years), and the like (Fig. 4).

Medical science is beginning to recognize its **limitations**. What happens after the miracles? What happens after the kidney transplants and the heart transplants? Everyone still eventually dies. There must be **a time to stop**—a time beyond which we are **causing more grief to the patient** by taking away their control, their dignity, and their finances.

By providing **excellent end-of-life care** we are **developing a new aphorism** that states our mission as:

New 21st century aphorism:
To cure when it is reasonable
To relieve symptoms often
To comfort always

REFERENCES

1. Doyle D, Hanks G, Cherny N, et al. Introduction. In: Doyle D, ed. *Oxford Textbook of Medicine.* 2nd ed. New York: Oxford University Press; pp.1–5.
2. Corr CA. Death in modern society. In: Doyle D, ed. *Oxford Textbook of Medicine.* 2nd ed. New York: Oxford University Press; 1998:33.

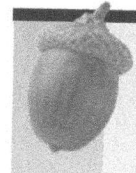

Historical Perspective
IN A NUTSHELL

Modern medicine has created a death from chronic disease by curing many of the causes of premature death.

Dying now takes much longer—an average of 30 months after a terminal diagnosis is established.

These changes have tremendous physical, social, and economic implications.

Cultural Diversity in End-of-Life Care

CHAPTER 5

Planning for Diverse Populations

The ethnic, cultural, and religious diversity that gives America its own unique background is also adding a new dimension to the special needs that health care practitioners must address when providing end-of-life care to members of these different communities. **Studies have shown that racial, ethnic, and gender groups differ significantly in end-of-life health care wishes** (1,2).

Reality—Ethnic minorities currently compose one third of the population of the United States!

Minorities are almost the majority!

When faced with difficult, complex, and multiple choices for health care treatment, patients and families draw on their inner resources, which may include cultural expectations of treatment, familial supports, and spiritual or religious beliefs. Along with these strengths patients and families may be faced with barriers to health care or treatment that may include lack of access as a result of language, education, economic deficits, or decreased formal and informal support systems.

Table 1 shows that end-of-life preferences by these groups may conflict with the way health care is provided in the United States.

Health care providers in the United States are accustomed to telling patients the truth about their conditions, but this may present some cultural conflict. For example, Arabs express reluctance to tell family members "bad news." They also avoid the use of the words "death" and "cancer."

Communication strategies to avoid cultural conflicts include:

- Be aware that a patient may want to know the truth but the patient's family wants to protect the same patient from the truth.

- Remember the obligation to tell the patient the truth, but be sensitive and communicate with the patient and family in the least threatening manner possible.

- Be careful not to generalize all individuals in a particular group.

TABLE 1

End-of-Life Preferences

	Arab Muslims		Arab Christians		Hispanics		Blacks		Whites	
	Male	Female	Male	Female	Male	Female	Male	Female	Male	Female
Believes family must care for dying individual	X	X	X	X						
Believes family should not care for dying individual							X	X	X	X
Prefers not to burden family at end of life (EOL)							X			
Prefers to die away from home, e.g., in nursing home							X	X		
Prefers to die at home	X	X	X	X					X	X
Is receptive to hospitals and hospice					X	X			X	X
Seeks to avoid nursing homes	X	X	X	X	X	X				
Is unfamiliar with concept of hospice	X	X	X	X						
Believes it is important to have advance directives									X	X
Requests no heroic measures be taken to extend life	X	X	X	X			X			
Prefers least medical intervention at EOL	X	X	X	X	X		X			
Prefers extensive medical intervention at EOL						X		X		

Source: Dr. Duffy and colleagues.

- Communicate openly with individual patients and their families to build understanding and trust.
- Inform patients and/or family members about advanced directives and ask patients which family members, if any, should be involved in treatment decisions.

Culturally competent care requires being flexible in communicating with patients. For example, providers might:

- Avoid using words such as "end-stage disease" or "dying" when communicating with patients who do not want to be told "bad news."

- A hospice nurse might need to refer to herself as "nurse" instead of "hospice nurse" when communicating with persons who are uncomfortable with that term.
- It is critical to be sensitive to patients' preferences while considering influences of race, ethnicity, and gender.

End-of-life preferences may be very specific to the intervention and vary between genders for the same ethnic group (2,3). For example:

- Hispanic females generally prefer extensive life-sustaining treatment, but are less likely to desire a feeding tube. In contrast, Hispanic men prefer the least medical intervention at the end of life.
- Arab and black men prefer no life-sustaining treatments, whereas black women favor extending life.

Gender differences within groups can present challenges for end-of-life decisions, especially because married women are often the surrogate decision makers for their husbands regarding end of life. Health care providers should encourage husbands and wives to discuss their end-of-life preferences while they are still healthy (2). Different groups have different preferences about the setting when they die (2). For example:

- Whites prefer to die at home, while blacks prefer dying away from home, such as at a nursing home.
- Arabs generally feel that the family should care for dying relatives and are less concerned about being a burden to their families.
- Arabs prefer to avoid nursing homes at the end of life and, in general, are unfamiliar with the concept of hospice.
- Hispanics also prefer to avoid nursing homes for dying, but are more receptive to hospitals and hospice.

Different groups also have different preferences about how much information they expect at the end of life. For example:

- Whites are generally very concerned about having choices related to their care.
- Whites desire details about what to expect physically during the dying process.
- Advanced directives are also important to whites.

REFERENCES

1. Searight HR, Gafford J. Cultural diversity at the end of life: issues and guidelines for family physicians. Am Fam Physician. 2005;71(3):515–522.
2. Duffy SA, Jackson FC, Schim SM, et al. Racial/ethnic preferences, sex preferences, and perceived discrimination related to end of life care. J Am Geriatr Soc. 2006;54:150–157.
3. O'Brien LA, Siegert EA, Grisso JA, et al. Tube feeding preferences among nursing home residents. J Gen Intern Med. 1997;12:364–371.

CHAPTER 6

African American Culture and End of Life

Active end-of-life care planning is not an unfamiliar concept to most African Americans. Providers who have these discussions, however, should remember a number of important cultural differences (1–4).

- Older African American adults might be reluctant to participate because of an understandable mistrust in the health care system based on past history of segregation and discrimination.
- **African Americans are less likely to complete advance directives such as do-not-resuscitate (DNR) orders or living wills.** They may feel that if they decided to opt for DNR, it would give the system the license to provide substandard care or give up on them "too soon."
- Religious beliefs may also play a role, in that many older African Americans believe that God is ultimately in control and is the only one who can determine the timing of death.

  Among both African American patients and physicians, more have been found to favor aggressive life-prolonging treatment in the case of terminal illness than among comparison white groups (1,3–5).

- Life support may be equated with life, and any effort at withholding life-sustaining therapies might be seen as another attempt of genocide by predominantly white institutions.
- Some request tube feeding even in the face of terminal illness, so providers should be very sensitive to issues regarding refusal or withdrawal of tube feedings.

  Communication about disease and prognosis is variable among African American families.

- Some families may request that certain diagnoses or disease prognoses be withheld from the patient to shelter them from disturbing information.
- Other patients and families favor forthright discussion of all medical issues and treatment plans.

- Some patients may prefer that their loved ones be the conduits for information. So direct provider-to-patient communication may be limited by patients' desire not to know the full implications of their illness.

> Remember: We are more alike than we are different!

The concept of family and loved ones may also vary among African Americans:

- Loved ones may be a patient's family members or *fictive kin*, people who are considered family as the result of long-standing relationships but may not be linked directly by blood ties.

- Fictive kin may be serving as the primary caregiver or even as the surrogate decision makers and may be sometimes more involved than the directly related family members.

    Extreme tact and sensitivity are called for when having discussions about advance care planning and end-of-life issues. Like Hispanics, African Americans prefer to make these decisions as a family (6,7).

    When providing care to African Americans, remember:

- They may not trust the health care system, especially regarding advanced directives and end-of-life care.

- Ensure that there is adequate time and the patient's family is present.

- Trust is critical in end-of-life care with African Americans and their families. Having established that trust before discussing or providing end-of-life care is often essential.

- Always ask the patient or family their understanding of the illness and treatment options, and use this as the basis for further discussion.

- Many African Americans have strong religious beliefs, and so having a trusted spiritual counselor as part of the team may be helpful for patients.

Death rituals for African Americans vary widely, perhaps because of the diversity in religious affiliations, geographic region, education, and economics (8–11). Differences include the following:

- Emotional expressions vary, with some African Americans crying and wailing while others are silent and stoic.

- Large gatherings and an expressed obligation to pay respects to the deceased are common.

- Southern and rural African Americans may maintain the custom of having the body at the house for the evening before the funeral. Family and friends gather at the house to help out where they can.

- Church members are especially helpful to the family during the viewing of the body and funeral.

- Strong religious beliefs—seeing the death as a reflection of God's will or plan, believing that the deceased is in God's hands, and being reunited in heaven after death—help many African Americans to grieve while maintaining a connection with the deceased.

- Bereaved African Americans are more likely to seek help from clergy than heath care professionals.

REFERENCES

1. Caralis P, Davis B, Wright K, et al. The influence of ethnicity and race on attitudes toward advance directives, life-prolonging treatments, and euthanasia. J Clin Ethics. 1993;4: 155–165.
2. Eleazer GP, Hornung C, Egbert CB, et al. The relationship between ethnicity and advance directives in a frail older population. J Am Geriatr Soc. 1996;44:938–943.
3. Hopp FP, Duffy S. Racial variations in end-of-life care. J Am Geriatr Soc. 2000;48: 658–663.
4. Mouton CP. Cultural and religious issues for African Americans. In: Braun KL, Pietsch JH, Blanchette PL, eds. *Cultural Issues in End-of-Life Decision Making*. Thousand Oaks, Calif: Sage; 2000.
5. Mebane EW, Oman RF, Kroonen LT, et al. The influence of physician race, age, and gender on physician attitudes toward advance care directives and preferences for end-of-life decision making. J Am Geriatr Soc. 1999;47:579–591.
6. Perkins HS, Geppert CMA, Gonzales A, et al. Cross-cultural similarities and differences in attitudes about advance care planning. J Gen Intern Med. 2002;17:48–57.
7. Waters CM. Understanding and supporting African Americans' perspectives on end-of-life care planning and decision making. Qual Health Res. 2001;11:385–398.
8. Perry HL. Mourning and funeral customs of African Americans. In: Irish DP, Lundquist KF, Nelsen VJ, eds. *Ethnic Variations in Dying, Death, and Grief*. Washington, DC: Taylor & Francis; 1993.
9. Hines Smith S. Now that mom is in the Lord's arms, I just have to live the way she taught me: Reflections on an elderly, African American mother's death. J Gerontol Soc Work. 1999;32:41–51.
10. Hines Smith S. Fret no more my child . . . for I'm all over heaven all day: religious beliefs in the bereavement of African American, middle-aged daughters coping with the death of an elderly mother. Death Stud. 2002;26:309–323.
11. Neighbors HW, Musick MA, Williams DR. The African American minister as a source of help for serious personal crises: bridge or barrier to mental health care? Health Educ Behav. 1998;25:759–777.

CHAPTER 7

Hispanic Views on Death and Dying

Provider and patient differences in culture, values, spiritual/religious, health beliefs, and worldviews can add to the complexity of end-of-life or health care decision making by Hispanic elders (1). In providing end-of-life care to Hispanics, providers should remember these issues of importance:

- Hispanics are more likely than whites to approve the use of cardiopulmonary resuscitation, hospitalization, the use of antibiotics, intubation, and intravenous nutrition.
- They are generally less comfortable discussing end-of-life issues compared to African Americans and whites.
- They are less likely to have an appointed health care proxy or written advanced health care directives, preferring to depend on available family members.

There are significant barriers to completion of an advanced care directive by Hispanics because of more distrust of physicians and the health care system. However, this tends to vary across Hispanic ethic groups with Mexican Americans being more trusting of their physicians and more likely to discuss advanced care planning with them (1).

The act of dying and death has been a more naturally accepted process culturally in the Hispanic communities than other communities (1). In this regard providers should expect the following:

- Religion, faith, and spirituality hold an important role in the acceptance of death.
- In discussing dying and death, Hispanics often incorporate *dichos*, or sayings, about God and their faith.

In contrast, although death appears to be more readily accepted by Hispanic older adults, the use of hospice services tends to be significantly lower for this group (1,2). Reasons for not using hospice services include the following:

- Lack of knowledge about hospice programs.
- The use of hospice services would denote "giving up hope and faith" in the life of the dying patient.
- Lack of insurance.
- Distrust in the provider or health care system.

Hispanics believe it is detrimental to patients to let them know about the seriousness of their illness in order to spare them unnecessary pain and that it is the family's obligation to take over control of the situation (1,3,4–6). In this regard, the provider should remember that:

- Hispanics, like African Americans, prefer to make advanced directive and end-of-life care decisions as a family.
- Hispanic older adults, in particular, do not make end-of-life decisions autonomously; rather, decisions are made in a familial context usually with reliance on the physician for guidance.

Hispanic death rituals are heavily influenced by Catholic beliefs where spirituality is very important (7,8). This perspective can be seen by the following:

- The belief that there is a continuing relationship between the living and the dead through prayer and visits to the grave.
- Grief is expressed by crying openly where women may wail loudly but men may act according to *machismo*, where there is a belief that men should act strong and not show overt emotion.
- There is a preference for burial rather than cremation.
- Novenas for 9 days.
- Mass for the deceased during the first year, then yearly.
- Family gatherings with food.
- Lighted candles.

Recommendations to providers for patient and family discussions on end-of-life decision making include the following:

- Assess the patient and family, when applicable, for understanding of end-of-life issues and values associated with making health care decisions.
- Become knowledgeable about the elder's cultural background; including social-historical, religion and spirituality, and health belief system.
- Recognize language issues and screen for barriers of service use.

- Use values history to process decisions and values related to medical care as a guide for provider and a method for Hispanic older adults and their families to begin to think about end-of-life issues.

- Conduct grassroots outreach efforts to discuss end-of-life issues.

- Recruit bilingual/bicultural volunteers in hospice and palliative care programs.

That which is not understood from the outside is usually understood when viewed from the inside.

REFERENCES

1. Talamantes MA, Gomez G, Braun KL. Advance directives and end-of-life care: The Hispanic perspective: In: Braun KL, Pietsch JH, Blanchette PL, eds. *Cultural Issues in End-of-Life Decision Making.* Thousand Oaks, Calif: Sage; 2000:83–100.
2. Talamantes MA, Lawler WR, Espino DV. Hispanic American elders: caregiving norms surrounding dying and the use of hospice services. Hosp J. 1995;10:35–49.
3. Rivera-Andino J, Lopez L. When culture complicates care. RN. 2000;63:47–49.
4. Perkins HS, Geppert CMA, Gonzales A, et al. Cross-cultural similarities and differences in attitudes about advance care planning. J Gen Intern Med. 2002;17,48–57.
5. Waters CM. Understanding and supporting African Americans' perspectives on end-of-life care planning and decision making. Qual Health Res. 2001;11:385–398.
6. Blackhall LJ, Murphy ST, Frank G, et al. Ethnicity and attitudes toward patient autonomy. JAMA. 1995;274:820–825.
7. Clements PT, Vigil GJ, Manno MS, et al. Cultural perspectives of death, grief, and bereavement. J Psychosoc Nurs. 2003;41:18–26.
8. Munet-Vilaro F. Grieving and death rituals of Latinos. Oncol Nurs Forum. 1998;25:1761–1763.

CHAPTER 8

Understanding the Jewish Culture

There are several major groups within Judaism, and the interpretation of Jewish law and practice may allow for wide variation in rituals (1). Providers should be aware of the following:

- Funerals are generally performed as soon after death as possible because there is a belief that the soul begins a turn to heaven immediately after death.
- There is also a belief that the body is a holy repository of the soul and should be treated and cared for with respect.
- A black ribbon or torn clothing symbolizing mourning or grief is worn by mourners.
- *Shiva* is the process of receiving guests during the grieving process.
- Families are cared for by their friends and the religious community while they contemplate their loss.
- Mourners may stay seated on low stools, mirrors may be covered, and mourners may perform only minimal amounts of grooming and/or bathing.
- Families may not place a headstone at the grave site until the first-year anniversary of the death coinciding with the end of the traditional year of mourning.
- There is a daily recitation of the *kaddish*, a life-affirming mourning prayer by mourners.
- Religious beliefs often change and observant people may become more or less observant when death occurs or may wish to break with tradition when faced with death.

REFERENCES

1. Clements PT, Vigil GJ, Manno MS, et al. Cultural perspectives of death, grief, and bereavement. J Psychosoc Nurs. 2003;41:18–26.

CHAPTER 9

Mourning in the Asian Culture

In the Asian culture, death—especially of an infant or child—is deeply mourned. There are a variety of traditions and beliefs concerning death within Asian culture (1–3), such as the following:

- Family members may wear white clothing or headbands for a period of time.
- Elaborate funeral ceremonies are the norm for marking the soul's passing to the afterlife.
- Sadness and grief may be expressed as somatic complaints because mental illness is often considered a disgrace to the family.
- **Buddhist belief uses death as an opportunity for improvement in the next life.** To enter death in a positive state of mind and surrounded by monk and family helps the deceased to become reborn on a higher level.
- Customs require a display of grief, wearing of traditional white cloth, openly showing grief, and even wailing at times.
- The body should be handled in a worthy and respectful way.

Hinduism is unique as a religion because its roots do not spring from a single scripture, founder, or sacred place but is seen as more of an umbrella term to describe a set of philosophies, cultures, and way of life. **However, the approach to death is fairly uniform because of the central belief in the laws of karma and reincarnation among all Hindus** (4,5). In general, providers should expect the following beliefs and rituals:

- Each birth is linked to actions taken in previous births.
- Births and deaths are part of a cycle that each person is seeking to transcend through the accumulation of good karmas (actions) ultimately leading to liberation of the soul.
- The body is bathed, massaged in oils, dressed in new clothes, and then cremated before the next sunrise to facilitate the soul's transition from this world to the next.

- Rituals are conducted for 10 days while the deceased member's soul watches over the family. On the 11th day, the soul releases its attachment to the former life.

> It's little wonder you Christians are afraid to die—it's like a hard test in school; you either **pass or fail!** I know I'm just coming back!"

REFERENCES

1. Lawson LV. Culturally sensitive support for grieving parents. Matern Child Nurs. 1990;15:76–79.
2. Dimond B. Disposal and preparation of the body: Different religious practices. Br J Nurs. 2004;13:547–549.
3. Truitner K, Truitner N. Death and dying in Buddhism. In: Irish DP, Lundquist KF, Nelsen VJ, eds. *Ethnic Variations in Dying, Death, and Grief.* Washington, DC: Taylor & Francis; 1993.
4. Clements PT, Vigil GJ, Manno MS, et al. Cultural perspectives of death, grief, and bereavement. J Psychosoc Nurs. 2003;41:18–26.
5. Spector R. *Cultural Diversity in Health & Illness.* 5th ed. Upper Saddle River, NJ: Prentice Hall Health; 2000.

CHAPTER 10

Death Practices in the Muslim Culture

In the Muslim culture, it is believed that at the time of death the soul is exposed to God. There is a belief about afterlife, and the Islamic religion dictates that the purpose of the worldly life is to prepare for the eternal life (1). The following rituals are important to Muslims:

- The dying patient should be positioned facing Mecca.
- The room is perfumed, and anyone who is unclean should leave the room.
- Passages from the Qur'an are read to the dying patient.
- Organ donation is permissible with family permission when a patient is determined to be brain dead.
- Family members prepare the body for burial following the pronouncement of death.
- Muslim culture does not encourage wailing, but crying is permissible.
- Personal prayers are recited while standing, but prayers from the Qur'an may not be recited near the corpse.
- Women are traditionally prohibited from visiting cemeteries.

REFERENCES

1. Ross H. Islamic tradition at the end of life. Medsurg Nurs. 2001;10:83–87.

CHAPTER 11

Building Cultural Bridges with Other Cultures

Patients make medical decisions based on cultural and religious needs. Those aspects must always be taken into account and those boundaries must be respected when we are discussing terminal illness and end-of-life care. Within the framework of a patient-centered approach, health care providers should discuss quality of life issues with their patients, as well as ultimately how they want to approach the end-of-life process.

With living in the United States comes a multitude of cultural attitudes and rituals regarding death, dying, and end-of-life health care issues that health care providers must consider. For example:

- Some West African cultures believe that telling a person they are very sick or dying is predicting the future—if you say something bad will happen, it will.
- In many cultures, it is believed that if the body is opened up for surgery there is a chance for evil spirits to enter the person.
- Latinos typically do not believe in nursing homes and tend to make their own care arrangements for terminally ill family members.
- European and African Americans generally believe a patient should be told the diagnosis of a terminal illness, whereas Korean and Hispanic Americans do not.

In addition to its cultural diversity, America has more religions and faith groups than can be calculated. And each of these groups has specific rituals and approaches to dealing with death and dying, such as the following:

- The Buddhist faith teaches that a person's state of mind while dying is of great importance. To help achieve a peaceful state of mind, the dying person is surrounded by family, friends, and monks who recite Buddhist scripture and mantras.
- Practicing Catholics who are dying let their relatives and friends know they wish to receive the last rites, which is usually accompanied by the sacrament of reconciliation and receiving holy communion as *viaticum*, or food for the journey.

- Islamic practices surrounding death vary, but generally the dying are positioned on their backs with their heads facing Mecca. The room is perfumed, and Islamic scriptures are read by the dying person or a relative.

- In the Hindu religion, at the time of death, holy ash must be applied to the forehead while holy mantras are chanted.

- Judaism mandates the body be treated with awe and reverence, and embalming or viewing of the body is usually not permitted because this tends to turn the person into an object.

Religious or spiritual beliefs can have a powerful impact on end-of-life care and the outcome for a dying patient. Providers need to be prepared for—and be open to—the spiritual and cultural differences of patients. Developing an approach to end-of-life care that respects patients and their families' requirements requires open dialogue among everyone involved. The following key areas should be addressed and considered by providers regarding cultural and spiritual sensitivity:

- Ask patients if they wish to receive information and make decisions for their own care, or if they prefer that their families handle such matters.

- If religion is an important part of the person's life, clergy members should be included in the discussions.

- Be straightforward with patients. Let them know that you will tell them what they want to know, and ask if you should talk to their family members or not.

- If there is a language barrier, an independent outside translator should be brought in, particularly if the burden of translating would otherwise fall on the shoulders of a young or adolescent family member.

In terms of determining spirituality, ask open-ended questions, such as "What gives you your strength?" or "What is the most meaningful thing in your life?"

Few people are ever offended by a statement such as "I know different people have very different ways of understanding illness and death. Please help me understand how you see things."

Regardless of the patient's ethnic background, religious affiliation, or cultural beliefs, each individual's situation truly is its own culture. **The end-of-life provider must always be sensitive to the issues at hand and then treat each case individually.** All people have their own unique beliefs and philosophy of how they will spend the last moments of their life.

REFERENCES

1. Brandhorst HW. Patterns in grief/loss/bereavement: a comparative ethnic study. Dissertation Abstracts International-B Series, 2000;60/09:4877.
2. Clements PT, Vigil GJ, Manno MS, et al. Cultural perspectives of death, grief, and bereavement. J Psychosoc Nurs. 2003;41:18–26.

3. Dimond B. Disposal and preparation of the body: different religious practices. Br J Nurs. 2004;13:547–549.
4. Perkins HS, Geppert CMA, Gonzales A, et al. Cross-cultural similarities and differences in attitudes about advance care planning. J Gen Intern Med. 2002;17:48–57.
5. Spector R. *Cultural Diversity in Health & Illness*. 5th ed. Upper Saddle River, NJ: Prentice Hall Health; 2000.

Approach to the Patient

CHAPTER 12

Delivering Bad News

No one enjoys giving bad news. However, there are proven methods that are more effective than winging it, as it were. Following these **guidelines** gives the health care provider **confidence** that they are doing the most professional job possible and provides the **most reliable possibility of acceptance** from the patient or his or her family.

Preparing to Give Bad News

- Choose a **quiet, comfortable** room where there will be **no interruptions**.
- Turn **off your beeper and cell phone**.
- Determine **who** is to be present—ask the patient if possible.
- Be sure to **review the medical information** and make sure it is accurate.
- Prepare for **special circumstances**: Patient is comatose, demented, can't understand or speak English.

COMMUNICATING THE BAD NEWS

Steps in Giving Bad News

- **Introduce yourself**, and have **others introduce themselves** and state their relationships to the patient.
- Determine **what the patient or family knows**: "What is your understanding of your present condition," or "What have the doctors told you?" Make no assumptions!
- Give a **"warning shot!"** "I'm afraid I have some bad news." Then **pause**.
- Present the bad news in a **direct and succinct manner**. Use **lay terms** so there is no misunderstanding.
- Then **sit quietly** for as long as it takes. (It may seem like an eternity!) **Wait** for the patient to respond and take your cue from that.
- If there is no response after a **prolonged silence**, you may gently say something like, "Tell me what you are thinking."
- Be **ready for emotions**—feeling angry, sad, numb, fearful, and so on.

- **Validate and normalize** those feelings. It's okay to interject personal statements if appropriate: "I lost my mother last year and know how you feel."

- **Answer questions** and provide information in small chunks. The discussion is like peeling an **onion**. Provide initial information and assess the patient or family's understanding. If they need more information, go to the next layer to meet their needs. Many people won't require a lot of details.

- Assess thoughts of **self-harm**.

- Provide a **follow-up plan**. This is very important as patient or family will have further questions once the information has "soaked in." "I'll be back in the morning—be sure to write down any questions that you might have."

- Offer to **involve others**—social work, chaplain, and so on (1).

FINAL COMMENT

Despite the challenges in giving a patient bad news, the health care provider can find **tremendous gratification** in **providing a therapeutic presence** during a patient's greatest time of need. A growing body of evidence demonstrates that the attitude and communication skills of the one delivering bad news plays a crucial role in how well patients accept and cope with the bad news (2,3).

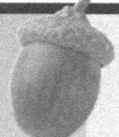

Delivering Bad News
IN A NUTSHELL

1. Have **accurate information**.
2. **Start with**: "What do you know about this condition?" or "What have other doctors told you?"
3. **Warning shot**: "I have some bad news!"
4. **State the bad news**: Use terms the patient will understand.
5. **WAIT; stop talking; be quiet!** (How long do you wait? My mentor says, "Until hell freezes over!")
6. **Follow** the patient's lead.
7. **End**: Always have a follow-up plan; "We will talk again this evening (tomorrow, in the morning)." Keep that follow-up time.

"What do you know?"

"Warning shot"

Give bad news.

Shut up and listen!

"Peel the onion": one layer of information at a time

Follow-up meeting

REFERENCES

1. Ambuel B. Giving bad and sad news. In: Weissman DE, Ambuel B, eds. *Improving End-of-Life Care: A Resource Guide for Physician Education.* Milwaukee: The Medical College of Wisconsin; 1999.
2. Vandekieft GK. Breaking bad news. Am Fam Physician. 2001;64:1975–1978.
3. Schmid MM, Kindlimann A, Langewitz W. Recipients' perspective on breaking bad news: how you put it makes a difference. Patient Educ Couns. 2005;58:244–251.

CHAPTER 13

The Family Conference

Just as in pediatrics, in palliative medicine we are often dealing with a lot of concerned people other than the patient. In fact, the patient is usually the easiest person to deal with. However, it is very important that all those concerned have a chance for input and their questions answered. One family member can derail all the best intentions. The following elements will ensure success (1–3).

> **Warning: Notify** out-of-town relatives ahead!

Before the Meeting
- Clarify the **goals** of the meeting in your own mind and in the minds of the other professionals who may be attending with you.
- Be sure everyone is on the **same page** before you talk to the family.
- Find a comfortable place that is **private** and **quiet**.
- **Circular seating** is preferred so everyone can face each other.

WHO ATTENDS THE "FAMILY" CONFERENCE?

Who Should Be There
- **Patient**, if able to participate. **Ask** the patient **who** they want present!
- **Legal decision maker** (designated power of attorney [DPOA])
- **Family members**
- **Social support** (friends, minister, others)
- Key **health care professionals**

Introductions
- Introduce **yourself** and other professionals.
- Have **family members** and others introduce themselves and explain their relationship to the patient.

- Set the **ground rules**: Each member will have a chance to ask questions and express their views; no interruptions are allowed.

Review the Medical Condition

- Determine what the family already knows: **"How do you think Grandma is doing?"** The answers to this question will quickly tell you if there is consensus and what the family's expectations are.
- Ask each family member if he or she has any questions about the medical condition.
- Defer any decisions to the next step.

WHO TALKS WHEN?

Discussion

- With a patient who can make decisions, have the patient speak first: **"What decisions are you considering?"**
- If the patient is not decisional, ask each family member, **"What do you think the patient would want if he or she could tell us?"**
- Try to always guide the discussion back to **"What would the patient want?"**

If There Is No Consensus

- Use **time as an ally**: "Think about what we have said, and we can talk again tomorrow."
- Emphasize that decisions should be based on **what the patient would want**.

KNOW WHEN TO STOP!

Ending the Meeting

- **Don't extend** the meeting indefinitely—everyone gets tired.
- **Restate the decisions** that were made so they are perfectly clear to everyone.
- If there is no consensus, state that there is **no clear consensus** and a follow-up meeting is to be scheduled, but restate the decision that needs to be made.
- Identify a **family spokesperson** for ongoing communications, if possible.
- **Thank everyone** for their time. Even if the meeting didn't go well, you will gain respect for next time by showing kindness.
- Go have a **stiff drink**!

After the Meeting

- **Document in the chart**: Who was present, what was discussed, the decisions that were made, and plans for follow up.
- **Be truthful** in the notes, but **never be disrespectful** to any family member and **never use any derogatory remarks** in charting. If there is bickering between family

members, just chart that "family could not agree" or "no consensus was reached." (Always remember your notes could be read in court!)

REFERENCES

1. Ambuel B. Conducting a family conference. In: Weissman DE, Ambuel B, eds. *Improving End-of-Life Care: A Resource Guide for Physician Education*. Milwaukee: The Medical College of Wisconsin; 1999.
2. Lang F, Quill T. Making decisions with families at the end of life. Am Fam Physician. 2004;70:719–23, 725–726.
3. Storey P, Knight C. *UNIPAC Five: Caring for the Terminally Ill—Communication and the Physician's Role on the Interdisciplinary Team*. New York: American Academy of Hospice and Palliative Medicine; 2003.

CHAPTER 14

Dealing with Anger

Elizabeth Kübler-Ross identified **anger** as a **predictable** part of the dying process expressed by seriously ill patients and their families. Most **health professionals**, confronted by the angry patient or family, either tend to **get angry** back or to **withdraw physically and psychologically** from the situation. Neither of these are helpful coping strategies (1).

UNDERSTANDING THE SOURCE OF ANGER

It is always helpful to remember the anger and hostility projected toward the health care worker is displaced (**transference**: "kill the messenger" type of reaction) (2).

Other sources of anger include the following:

- **"Rational anger"**—a genuine insult (e.g., waiting 6 hours to see the doctor or for pain medications to arrive)
- **Organic pathology**—cerebral metastasis, frontal lobe lesion, dementia, or delirium.
- **Personality style/disorder**—this person has always approached life via anger or mistrust.

In end of life, **fear** is the most common **source of anger**:

- Fear of pain or suffering
- Fear of the unknown (death)
- Fear of losing control of bodily functions or cognition
- Fear of becoming a burden on the family
- Fear of dying alone
- Fear of unfinished physical or spiritual business

APPROACH TO ANGER

Anger can be directed **internally** (e.g., "I didn't take care of myself," or "I shouldn't have smoked," etc.). This type of internal anger may lead to depression, anxiety, or withdrawal. **Outward anger** is often directed at health care workers, the hospital, family members, or God. As a result, health professionals often avoid engaging and empathizing with these patients. Research shows that when this happens, the dying patient may not get adequate analgesia or emotional support and may suffer unnecessarily (3).

Here are some helpful **approaches to dealing with outward anger**:

- **Never get angry at the patient**!
- Practice active and sympathetic **listening**—let patients vent and try to understand their story and their situation.
- **Name the emotion**: "You seem very angry . . .?"
- **Validate** patients' feelings so they know you are listening. "If I were in your situation, I would certainly feel upset." (This is much better than taking ownership of the patient's anger by saying something like "I feel bad for you!" Now there is confusion about who is taking on the emotional work—it needs to be the patient!) (4). Acknowledging the patient's right to feel angry starts the healing process and builds a therapeutic relationship.
- **Never argue**—it is counterproductive.
- Explore their **fears**: "Tell me what frightens you."
- **Normalize** the anger: "What you are feeling is normal!"
- Display **empathy and concern**, but avoid empty statements like "I know what you are going through" (unless you really do!). **Paraphrasing the patient's comments** will show you are listening and trying to understand; "So you feel it is so unfair that you have this terminal disease when you always tried to take care of yourself!"

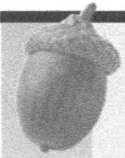

Dealing with Anger
IN A NUTSHELL

Never get angry yourself—you are most likely not the source of their anger.

Listen!

Name the emotion: "You seem angry. . . ."

Validate the patient's feelings: "I'd probably be angry too if . . ."

Never argue!

Define the patient's fears.

Let the patient know **anger is a normal** part of the grieving process.

Display genuine **empathy and concern**.

REFERENCES

1. Wang-Cheng B. Dealing with anger. In: Weissman DE, Ambuel B, eds. *Improving End-of-Life Care: A Resource Guide for Physician Education.* Milwaukee: The Medical College of Wisconsin; 1999.
2. Bell HS. Curbside consultation—a potentially violent patient? Am Fam Physician. 2000;61:2237–2238.
3. Manetto C, McPherson S. The behavioral-cognitive model of pain. Clin Geriatr Med. 1996;12:461–472.
4. Houston RE. The angry dying patient, primary care companion. J Clin Psychiatry. 1999;1:5–8.

CHAPTER **15**

The Spiritual Assessment

When we stand with patients as they face the end of their life, we are in a position to help them address some of life's (and medicine's) greatest mysteries. Something programmed into the human mind causes us to question our existence and what becomes of us after death (1). As professionals we must recognize the importance of this spirituality in our patient's physical and emotional well-being while maintaining an open-minded, balanced approach to their medical care without compromising scientific integrity. Tremendous spiritual growth often occurs when we face our mortality (Table 2).

SPIRITUALITY VS. RELIGION

Although many people use the terms **spirituality** and **religion** interchangeably, they are in fact **very different**. **Spirituality** is the broad, complex, multidimensional, mysterious part of human experience that includes the search for meaning, purpose,

TABLE 2

Importance of Spirituality

95% of Americans believe in God (or a supreme power).	Gallup G. *Religion in America 1990*. Princeton, NJ: Princeton Religious Center; 1990.
96% of physicians believe spiritual well-being is important to health.	Koenig HG, Oyama O. Religious beliefs and practices in family medicine. Arch Fam Med. 1998;7:431–435.
77% of patients would like for their health-care provider to consider their spiritual needs as part of their medical care.	Maugans TA, Wadland WC. Religion and family medicine: a survey of physicians and patients. J Fam Pract. 1991;32:210–213.
80% of patients report that doctors or nurses never or rarely discuss spiritual issues with them.	Levin JS, Larson DB, Puchalshi CM. Religion and spirituality in medicine: research and education. JAMA. 1997;278:792–793.

42

and truth in life. Human spirituality is the huge umbrella of the unknown that includes our inner belief systems and how we make sense of the events in our lives.

Religion attempts to answer our spiritual questions by providing a specific set of beliefs, teachings, rules, and practices. There is one human spirit but many religions. Many people find spirituality through religion; however, some find spirituality through communing with nature, music, the arts, the quest for scientific truth, or a set of values and principles (2).

Everyone has a human spirit, but not everyone is religious; **nor is religion a requirement for spirituality**. A person may not practice a specific religion but still have spiritual needs that should be met.

TAKING A SPIRITUAL HISTORY

Some type of spiritual history should be taken on all end-of-life patients. Knowing a person's spiritual strength or distress reflects his or her health and response to medical care, either in a positive or negative manner.

INFORMAL SPIRITUAL ASSESSMENT

Look for **visual clues** of the patient's spirituality in the home, hospital room, or on the body (jewelry, etc):

- Cross, Bible, Qur'an, crucifix, paintings, or other religious symbols
- Prayer beads, pins, jewelry
- Religious leader's card, church newsletters, or other literature
- What they are watching on TV or music they are listening to

    Listen closely for **verbal clues**:

- Patient refers to God or a Higher Power ("Friend," "Savior," "Parent," "Man upstairs")
- Statements such as these:
    - "People are praying for me." (community support)
    - "It's all in God's hands now." (trust)
    - "Why is God letting this happen to me?" (anger)
    - Listen for metaphorical language and themes in their stories, such as searching for meaning or fear of the unknown.
- References to church, prayer, and so on

FORMAL SPIRITUAL ASSESSMENT

One method (there are others) of formal spiritual assessment is the **HOPE questions** (see Table 2). These questions have not been validated by research but have proven to be clinically useful in opening discussions about spiritual issues.

The HOPE approach does not immediately focus on the word *spirituality* or *religion*, which minimizes barriers to discussion based on language. It also allows those for whom religion is important to volunteer that information. The questions can be asked in many ways. Table 3 provides several examples.

> **Remember: Spiritual pain is more devastating than the most vile of physical afflictions!**

TABLE 3

Examples of Questions for the HOPE Approach to Spiritual Assessment

H: Hope Sources of hope, meaning, comfort, strength, peace, love, and connection

- "We have been discussing your support systems. I was wondering, what is there in your life that gives you internal support?"
- "What are your sources of hope, strength, comfort, and peace?"
- "What do you hold on to during difficult times?"
- "What sustains you and keeps you going?"
- "For some people, their religious or spiritual beliefs act as a source of comfort and strength in dealing with life's ups and downs; is this true for you?"

  If the answer is "Yes," go on to "O" and "P" questions.
  If the answer is "No," consider asking, "Was it ever?" If "Yes," "What changed?"

O: Organized Religion

- "Do you consider yourself part of an organized religion?"
- "How important is this to you?"
- "What aspects of your religion are helpful and not so helpful to you?"
- "Are you part of a religious or spiritual community?" "Does it help you?" "How?"

P: Personal Practices

- "Do you have personal spiritual beliefs that are independent of organized religion?" "What are they?"
- "Do you believe in God?" "What kind of relationship do you have with God?"
- "What aspects of your spirituality or spiritual practices do you find most helpful to you personally?" (e.g., prayer, meditation, reading scripture, attending religious services, listening to music, hiking, communing with nature)

E: Effects on Medical Care and End-of-Life Issues

- "Has being sick affected your ability to do the things that usually help you spiritually (or affected your relationship with God?)"
- "Is there anything that I can do to help you access the resources that usually help you?"
- "Are you worried about any conflicts between your beliefs and your medical situation/care/decisions?"
- "Would it be helpful for you to speak to a clinical chaplain/community spiritual leader?"
- "Are there any specific practices or restrictions that I should know about in providing your medical care?" (e.g., dietary restrictions, use of blood products)

Reproduced and adapted with permission from Anandarajah G, Hight E. Spirituality and medical practice: using the HOPE questions as a practice tool for spiritual assessment. Am Fam Physician, 2001; 63: 81 to 88.

EFFECTS OF SPIRITUAL ASSESSMENT ON MEDICAL MANAGEMENT

Now what? Some feel comfortable dealing with spiritual issues, but remember we can go only as far with patients on their spiritual journey as we have gone on our own spiritual journey. We must guard against forcing our values on a vulnerable patient. Instead, our focus is on identifying and meeting the spiritual needs that in turn affect the patient's response to medical care.

General Spiritual Care

- Communicate effectively: Listen!
- Compassion and caring
- Encouragement of realistic hope
- Caring presence: Just be there!

Specialized Spiritual Care

- Often requires a professional spiritual leader—refer to a chaplain, minister, priest, rabbi, or other spiritual leader.
- We quickly refer to the cardiologist for a heart problem or the orthopedist for a bone problem. Why not refer as quickly to the chaplain for a spiritual concern?

WARNING

As we approach the very personal area of spirituality professionally, we must maintain the utmost respect for the patient's rights to autonomy and freedom of thought and belief. **Our personal spiritual beliefs** are generally **not relevant**. When

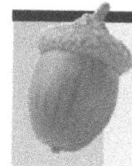

Spiritual Assessment
IN A NUTSHELL

Spirituality is often overlooked but is an **important part** of patient care.

Spirituality and religion are not the same thing!

Some type of **spiritual assessment** should be done on all patients in end-of-life care:

   Informal—Visual or verbal clues

   Formal—HOPE Questions

Assessing spiritual concerns has a **positive effect** on caregiver rapport and often helps patients cope with difficult times.

Remain **balanced** and open minded; affirm the patient's beliefs, enabling patients to claim what has encouraged them in life's journey.

Guard against forcing your values on a vulnerable patient.

Be quick to refer spiritual issues to the appropriate spiritual professional.

patients ask about our beliefs, it may indicate weakness or searching in their own beliefs. It is therefore **more therapeutic** not to just give opinions immediately but to ask, "Often, when patients ask about my beliefs, it tells me they are concerned about something. Can you tell me more about your concerns?" **If we simply explain our own religious beliefs to a patient, we may inadvertently rob them from their own journey to meaning** (3).

REFERENCES

1. Benson H. *Timeless Healing—the Power and Biology of Belief.* New York: Fireside; 1997.
2. Anandarajah G, Hight E. Spirituality and medical practice: using the HOPE questions as a practical tool for spiritual assessment. Am Fam Physician. 2001;63:81–88.
3. Storey P, Knight CF. *UNIPAC Two: Alleviating Psychological and Spiritual Pain in the Terminally Ill.* New York: American Academy of Hospital and Palliative Care; 2003:70–72.

CHAPTER 16

Giving Realistic Hope

One of the most difficult balances to maintain while caring for patients at the end of life is trying to be **realistic about their prognosis** but at the same time not taking away all their **hope** (the frame within which they construct their future). Medical professionals rightfully struggle to **promote hope and a positive outlook** in patients with advanced disease (1). Therefore we often fear that by telling someone the truth about their diagnosis, we become responsible for destroying hope.

The conflict between **truth telling and fear of destroying hope** often leads health professionals to convey overly optimistic prognoses or not to give this information at all (2). This behavior, although intended to protect the patient (and ourselves), is often perceived by patients and families as a feeling that "they are not telling me everything." Thus the very situation that we are trying to prevent is occurring because of the corrosive lack of trust and hope in the provider–patient relationship.

On the other side, we must deal with our **own biases**. Health professionals also want to hope for the best. We went into medicine hoping to cure disease, make patients feel better, and relieve suffering. Patients and families are often grateful to professionals that hold out hope. However, we have an **obligation to scientific integrity and must balance facts with realistic hope**.

HOPE AND TRUTH TELLING

Hope is a critical element for coping with advanced disease (3). However, truth telling does not necessarily rob patients of hope (2). Health care providers must realize that it is not their job to "correct" the patient's hope. The key question is **whether their hope is helping them cope effectively or whether it is interfering with appropriate planning and behavior**. When we talk to patients and **really listen** to them, we can almost always give them some **realistic assurances**.

Here are some factors that increase hope:

- Feeling valued
- Having meaningful relationships
- Honesty

- Humor
- Reminiscence
- Realistic goals (short, medium and, perhaps, long term)
- Pain and symptom relief

Factors that destroy hope include the following:

- Abandonment: "There is nothing else we can do" (there may be nothing to do to cure the disease, but there is **always something you can do for the patient!**).
- Isolation
- Lack of direction or goals
- Unrelieved pain and discomfort
- Dishonesty
- Feeling devalued or worthless

REDIRECTING GOALS

Redirecting patients' goals toward realistic hope seems to be important in their coping abilities, even though no studies have really examined how realistic hope might affect medical outcomes such as quality of life, survival, symptom management, or quality of death.

The goal of "cure" may need to be transitioned into a more **realistic goal** of "seeing my granddaughter graduate," "celebrating my 50th anniversary," "welcoming the new baby into the family," or even having a prepared and comfortable death.

Here are some questions that **initiate discussions** about redirecting goals:

- "Do you have long-term hopes and dreams that have been threatened by this illness?"
- "I too hope this disease will stay in remission, but if it doesn't, what other shorter-term goals might we work on together?"
- "We've been talking about treatments that are really not going to be effective, and we can't recommend those to you. But there are a lot of things we can still do to help you—let's focus on those."
- "What sorts of things do you have that are undone? Let's talk about how we might be able to make these happen."

HOPE FOR THE BEST, BUT PREPARE FOR THE WORST

Hoping for the best possible outcome while preparing the patient for the worst are not mutually exclusive strategies (4). It is reasonable for patients and families to **prepare for a range of outcomes**. There is no harm in making a living will, naming a health care proxy, addressing relationship concerns, and preparing financial matters, even while hoping for a cure or a miracle. Some patients may be more comfortable with this approach, especially early on in the course of a disease.

An approach to begin dialogue about "hoping for the best but preparing for the worst" might be to ask questions like these:

- "Have you thought about what might happen if things don't go the way we hope they will? Sometimes having a plan that prepares you for the worst makes it easier to focus on what you hope for most!"
- "Preparing for the worst doesn't mean we are giving up on you; it helps us arrange the best care, no matter what happens."
- "Thinking about the worst is often hard. What makes it hard for you to think about—what fears and concerns do you have?"

IMPARTING TRUE HOPE

Being able to impart true hope is fundamental to helping people at the end of life. Characteristics of a skilled end-of-life professional include the following (5):

- Honesty
- Forthrightness
- Confidence
- Good listening skills
- Calm demeanor
- Maintaining good eye contact with the patient
- Compassion
- Ability to allay fears and anxiety

> **We can all truthfully assure our patients that there can always be improvement in well being, even in the setting of the most deadly illness—and that is hope.**

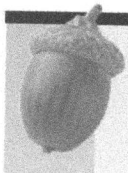

Hope
IN A NUTSHELL

The problem: Providing a patient scientific truth about their poor prognosis without destroying hope.

Never say, "There is nothing more we can do!" There is always something you can do for the patient, even if you can't cure the disease!

Redirect goals: "Do you have some special events coming up? Let's focus on your goals for them."

"Hope for the best, but prepare for the worst."

Be a good listener: When we truly understand, we can always provide some true reassurance.

REFERENCES

1. Butow PN, Dowsett S, Hagerty R, et al. Communicating prognosis to patients with metastatic disease: what do they really want to know? Support Care Cancer. 2002;10:161–168.
2. Tulsky JA. Beyond advanced directives: importance of communication skills at the end-of-life, JAMA. 2005;294:359–365.
3. Herth K. Fostering hope in terminally ill people. J Adv Nurs. 1990;15:1250–1259.
4. Back AL, Arnold RM, Quill TE. Hope for the best, and prepare for the worst. JAMA. 2003;138:439–443.
5. Groopman J. *The Anatomy of Hope: How People Prevail in the Face of Illness.* New York: Random House; 2004.

CHAPTER 17

The DNR or AND Discussion in Seriously Ill Patients

Many hospitals, hospices, long-term care facilities, and other medical facilities are transitioning from the DNR (Do Not Resuscitate) order to the AND (Allow Natural Death) order. The "Not" or negativism in DNR seems to confuse patients and their families into thinking that care for their loved one will be abandoned and all treatment stopped.

However, an order to Allow Natural Death (AND) is positive. It relays the information to the patient, to the family, and to the staff that the patient is dying and we will do all we can to allow that to happen naturally, without aggressive interference. Rather than implying withholding care (DNR), we are now acknowledging the completion of the cycle that is the miracle of life and death.

Both terms, *DNR* and *AND*, basically mean it is time to change the goal of treatment to palliation and cardiopulmonary resuscitation (CPR) is not appropriate. However, to patients and family members who are emotionally—not clinically—involved in this situation, AND seems a gentler, more positive approach.

AND is not accepted in all facilities yet, and it may be misunderstood until everyone is familiar with the terminology. If writing AND, be sure it is clear to everyone what is being ordered (1).

MEDICAL INFORMATION

Before an AND (DNR) discussion can take place, we must know the medical data that define outcomes of CPR in different populations.

Public's Expectations of CPR

- Television codes are 75% to 100% successful without sequelae (2).

- "Go ahead and bring me back once—then I'll decide if I like it or not!"

Truth about CPR

- Hospitalized patients: Survival to discharge is consistently reported as between 13% and 15% (3,4).

- Elderly patients with serious illnesses: Survival to discharge is less than 5% (2).

- Long-term care patients: Survival over 48 hours is consistently between 0% to as high as 3% (5).

Complications of CPR

- Chest trauma (fractured ribs, pneumothorax, etc.): 75%
- Aspiration: 25% to 50%
- Pain; loss of dignity

STARTING THE DISCUSSION

- Allow time: This discussion cannot be rushed.
- Sit down next to the patient in private area.
- Start with something like this: "I'd like to visit with you about some health care decisions that we will need to make in the future."

WHAT DOES THE PATIENT UNDERSTAND AND EXPECT?

- It is important to get the patient talking. Use open-ended sentences: "What is your understanding of this condition?" or "What have the doctors told you?"
- The patient's answer to these questions will immediately let you know if you have an easy job or a tough job ahead! If the patient has no understanding or an unrealistic view, then it is time to review data before going on. You may need to allow time for acceptance and come back later.
- Ask the patient to consider the future: "What goals do you have for the time you have left?" Now listen! Most patients with advanced disease have already thought a lot about dying—now they have a chance to express those thoughts.
- Validate and clarify what the patient says: "I think you are right that you will eventually die from this disease. What I hear you saying is that you want to be comfortable when that time comes."
- If possible, ask the patient to explain the values that have led them to their decisions: "Why do you feel that way?"

DISCUSS THE AND/DNR ORDER

- Use language the patient will understand and give it in small pieces.
- Start general and get more specific if the patient requests it.
- Never say, "Do you want us to do everything?" *Everything* is easily misinterpreted and hard to define.
- Use the phrase, "If you die in spite of our treatment, do you want us to attempt to bring you back?" Using the *die* word emphasizes the seriousness of CPR.
- If the patient agrees, tell him or her you will write an "Allow Natural Death" or DNR order in the chart.

CLARIFY FUTURE PLANS

- "We have decided on a DNR/AND order, but we will continue maximal medical therapy to meet your goals. Let's talk about those goals . . ."
- Never imply "There is nothing else to do!" There may not be anything to do to cure the disease, but there is much to do for the patient!
- This may be a great time to talk about palliative care or hospice referral also (6).
- **Know the medical facts**: about the patient and about CPR.

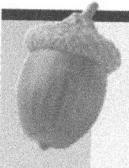

AND/DNR Orders in Seriously Ill Patients
IN A NUTSHELL

- **Know the medical facts**: about the patient and about CPR.
- Find out **what the patient understands and expects**: "What have you been told about your condition/your mother's condition?"
- **Listen carefully**: You won't be successful if you do all the talking! Ask open-ended questions.
- Discuss the specific **AND/DNR order**. Use the word *die* to emphasize CPR is serious. "If you die, do you want us to try to bring you back?"
- Give only the information that the patient asks for, in small chunks. Most health care professionals get too technical about CPR. Generally patients believe results of CPR are much better than they actually are—and that information may need to be shared.
- Discuss **future plans**: Emphasize that we are not abandoning the patient and that palliative care is not "No Care." It may be more care!
- **Write the order** in the chart and document the discussion you have had and who was present.

REFERENCES

1. Meyer C. New designation for allowing a natural death ("AND") would eliminate confusion and suffering when patients are resuscitated against their wishes. Hospice Patients Alliance. Available at: http://www.hospicepatients.org/and.html. Accessed February 19, 2006.
2. Diem SJ, Lantos JD, Tulsky JA. Cardiopulmonary resuscitation on television. Miracles and misinformation. N Engl J Med. 1996;334:1578–1582.
3. Education for Physicians on End-of-Life Care Trainer's Guide. Module 11, withholding, withdrawing therapy. In: Emanuel LL, von Gunten CJ, Ferris FD, eds. *Education for Physicians on End-of-Life Care/Institute for Ethics at the American Medical Association.* Chicago: EPEC Project, The Robert Wood Johnson Foundation; 1999.
4. The Support Principle Investigators. A controlled trial to improve care for seriously ill hospitalized patients. The study to understand prognosis and preferences for outcomes and risks or treatments (SUPPORT). JAMA. 1996;275:1232.
5. Finucane TE, Harper GM. Attempting resuscitation in nursing homes: policy considerations. J Am Geriatr. 1999;47:1261–1264.
6. von Gunten CF, Weissman DE. Discussing DNR orders in the hospital setting. *Fast Facts and Concepts.* Milwaukee: Medical College of Wisconsin; 2002.

CHAPTER 18

Advanced Directives in Health Care

Health care professionals have a duty to honor their patient's wishes concerning end-of-life choices (1). An advanced directive is any decision that patients make in advance concerning what they would want done to them if they are unable to make decisions in the future.

These may be expressed directly or by means of a proxy (Fig. 5).

INSTRUCTIVE OR "LIVING WILL"

The living will is a type of instructive advanced directive in which patients describe the type of treatment they wish to receive if they can no longer make decisions.

Advantages of the Living Will

- It names specific procedures or treatments that a patient does or does not want.

- It gives the health care team an idea of what the patient wants.

Disadvantages of the Living Will

- It does *not* provide for someone else to make medical decisions.

- Living wills are often vague, using phrases such as "No extraordinary means," No heroic measures," or "If I have no chance of normal recovery!" These terms are often subjective.

- It is also difficult to include in a living will all the possibilities that one might face in the future (e.g., new technologies or decisions that we could not anticipate).

PROXY OR DURABLE POWER OF ATTORNEY FOR HEALTH CARE

The durable power of attorney (DPOA) allows the designation of a surrogate medical decision maker of the patient's choosing. This surrogate decision maker makes medical care decisions for the patient in the event the patient is incapacitated.

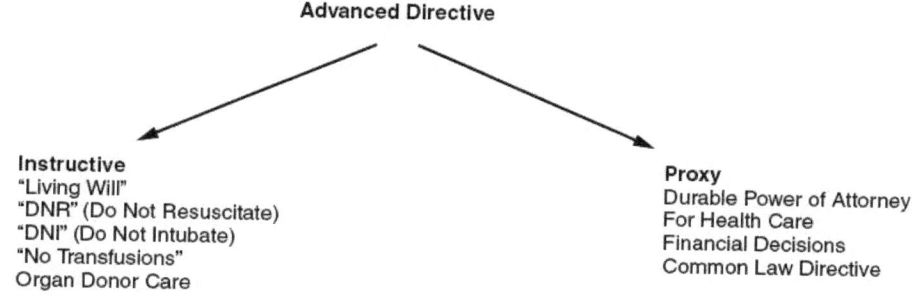

FIGURE 5 ● Common types of advanced directives.

Advantages of the DPOA

- Not all possible medical interventions need to be listed as in the living will: The DPOA can make reasonable decisions as they come along.

Disadvantages of the DPOA

- Patients have less control. They must trust their proxy to make the decisions that they would want made.

- The DPOA must be updated and kept current. For example, the original DPOA may no longer be able or available to serve in that capacity.

> **Important Point:** No advanced directive is in effect if the patient is decisional!

> **Corollary:** Everyone has the right to make *stupid* decisions!

WHO CAN BE NAMED AS THE DPOA?

Any competent adult can be named as DPOA! Most often patients select a family member or friend. However, the patient's choice should consent to being the DPOA—no sports heroes or movie stars without their consent!

WHEN TO DISCUSS AN ADVANCED DIRECTIVE

Advanced directives should be discussed with patients long before they are needed. Having that discussion during routine physicals or health maintenance examinations is ideal. In reality, however, certainly patients with any advanced disease should be approached about this form of "advanced disease planning."

LEGAL ISSUES

All 50 states recognize some form of DPOA. Federal enactment of the Patient Self-Determination Act (1990) requires that all patients be informed about their right to participate in health care decisions, including the right to have an advance directive (1). Advanced directives are legally binding in all 50 states.

HOW CAN PATIENTS PREPARE AN ADVANCE DIRECTIVE?

- Use a form provided on the Internet or from a hospital, hospice, or doctor's office. Forms for all 50 states are available at http://www.uslivingwillregistry.com/forms.shtm (2).

- Write their wishes themselves (letter or list) and sign it. It is better if it can be notarized or witnessed.

- Have a lawyer do it (not necessary unless complicated).

- A copy should be given to the doctor and patient's family. The physician is responsible to note "Advanced Directive" on the patient's chart.

- A copy should be provided to the hospital on any hospital admission.

CHANGING AN ADVANCED DIRECTIVE

Any advanced directive can be changed at any time. However, be sure the patient destroys the old form and provides the new form to all the appropriate people.

LIMITATIONS AND CHALLENGES

The current advance care process has many limitations, including the fact that most patients have not completed any type of advanced directive (3). Physicians often do not discuss end-of-life issues or DNR orders even when their patients have serious medical illnesses (4). Documents that are prepared are often misplaced, out of date, or the advanced directives are simply not followed.

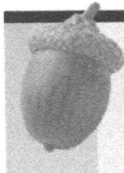

Advanced Directives
IN A NUTSHELL

- Promotion of advanced directives is a dominant strategy to improve end-of-life care.

- Advanced Directives should be discussed with patients before they are needed.

- Instructive Advanced Directives include living wills, or any other form of instruction that a patient leaves.

- Proxy Advanced Directive chooses someone else to make decisions when the patient cannot.

REFERENCES

1. Patient Self-Determination Act 1990. 42 USC 139 cc(a). Available at: http://caselaw .lp.findlaw.com/scripts/getcase.pl?court=9th&navby=case&no+9435534&exact=1. Accessed February 18, 2006.
2. US Living Will Registry. Available at: http://www.uslivingwillregistry.com/forms.shtm. Accessed February 18, 2006.
3. Crane MK, Wittink M, Doukas DJ. Respecting end-of-life treatment preferences. Am Fam Physician. 2005;72:1263–1270.
4. Teno JM, StevensM, Spernak S, et al. Role of written advance directives in decision making: insights from qualitative and quantitative data. J Gen Intern Med. 1998;13:439–446.

CHAPTER 19

Decision-Making Ability

Informed consent is based on the ethical principle that patients should be allowed to make decisions for themselves. However, in palliative care, there is often a point where a patient is no longer able to make their own decisions, and a surrogate or proxy decision maker is needed. Determining if a patient is decisional is often an issue.

PATIENT AUTONOMY

Both legally and ethically, Western culture favors an individual patient's right of self-determination (1). In other words, patients have a right to make poor choices as long as they are decisional. Restricting autonomy in our society requires convincing evidence that the patient's decision in unintended and will cause irreparable harm. Therefore, a patient is presumed to have decision-making capacity until proven otherwise (2)!

DEFINITIONS

Competency: This is a **legal term!** Medical professionals do not determine competency—only a judge! Don't use the term *competent* in a medical context.

Capacity: The patient's decision-making ability.

Decisional: A better word to use because it is less likely to get confused with the legal term *competency*.

For a patient to be decisional, three things are required:

1. The patient must be able to take in information. This ability is not limited to verbal or written information, but includes any alternative methods whereby a patient can take in information.

2. The patient must be able to process information that is **pertinent to the situation** (see "Decisional Thresholds" later).

3. The patient must be able to give back information (communicate his or her decisions).

TIME SPECIFIC

Decision-making capacity may be temporary or permanent. It may also fluctuate from hour to hour. Therefore, truly decisional patients should have **consistency** in their decisions (3). It helps to ask, "Can you repeat to me what we have just decided?" Or, "Tell me again what the consequences of this decision mean."

Patients who change their answer each time they are asked are suspect. The specific decision should seem consistent with the patient's previous values.

DECISIONAL THRESHOLDS

Here is the **tricky part**. Some decisions are more complex than others. Deciding if patients are decisional requires weighing the degree of their decision-making ability against the risks and benefits of the decision. For example a patient with moderate Alzheimer's disease who develops chest pain may be able to understand the need for antibiotics to fight pneumonia, but he or she may not be able to process the information about the risks and benefits of cardiac catheterization and angioplasty for coronary artery disease. They may be decisional on what to order for lunch but not decisional on which stock to trade in their portfolio!

A more complex decision (subjective) requires a higher level of decision-making ability. Many experts believe in a sliding scale view of decisionality. A higher level of certainty is needed when the decision poses greater harm or risk (4).

PITFALLS

Severe depression, hopelessness, or psychiatric diagnoses can make it difficult to interpret decisionality. Is the logic that the patient used to arrive at the decision logical? If they are making this decision because "aliens" told them to, we may want to question it. The question to ask yourself is "Are the patient's values speaking, or is it the underlying physical or mental illness?"

Complex cases should have consultation from a psychiatrist or the ethics committee.

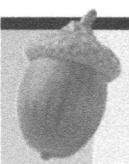

Decision-Making Ability
IN A NUTSHELL

Decision-making ability is a **gatekeeper**—patients who have it can make decisions for themselves; those who don't need a surrogate.

Patients are **considered decisional until proven otherwise!**

Competency is a **legal term**—not medical; use "capacity" or "decisional."

A decisional patient can **take in information, process the information** appropriately, and **give back information.**

The more **complex** the decision, the **higher level of decision-making ability** is required **(sliding scale).**

Severe **depression or mental illness complicates** determining decisional ability.

REFERENCES

1. Beauchamp TL, Childress JF. *Principles of Biomedical Ethics*. 4th ed. New York: Oxford University Press; 1994.
2. Storey P, Knight CF. *Ethical and Legal Decision Making When Caring for the Terminally Ill*. 2nd ed. New York: American Academy of Hospice and Palliative Medicine; 2003:25–33.
3. Arnold R. Decision making capacity. *Fast Facts*. Milwaukee: The Medical College of Wisconsin. Available at: http://www.eperc.mcw.edu/fastFact/ff_55.htm. Accessed February 23, 2006.
4. Tunzi M. Can the patient decide? Evaluating patient capacity in practice. Am Fam Physician. 2001;64:299–306.

CHAPTER 20

Goal Setting

Goal setting is the **most important part of palliative care**. Once a patient's, or family's, goals are clear, treatment becomes much more obvious. Remember, in palliative care the main focus should be on **quality of life**.

Often we approach patients with a choice of "treatment" or "treatment withdrawal." Here, treatment withdrawal is a negative choice. Rather, it is better to start the conversation as a patient-focused **positive decision**, such as "How can we help you live well for the time that is remaining?"(1)

> "Dude, why are you spending time tying down the deck chairs on the *Titanic*?"

"Living Well" in These Kinds of Situations

- Soon after a **life-limiting** diagnosis is made (e.g., cancer, stroke, congestive heart failure [CHF], chronic obstructive pulmonary disease [COPD], etc.)

- Outpatients with a stable **chronic disease**, as part of their advanced disease planning discussion

- **Healthy individuals** at their routine exams, as part of the advanced directive discussion

Who Is Involved

- The **decisional patient** (If there is a question about whether the patient is decisional, see Chapter 19 on decision-making capacity.)

- **Physician/health care provider** of record

- **Others**: family, friends, minister, and so on. Remember the goals should be set according to what the **patient** wants.

Starting the Discussion

- Express an **interest** and **need to comprehend** the patient's situation, understanding, and desires.

- Determine **what the patient knows**: Do not make any assumptions:
  - **"What have you been told** about your condition?"
  - **"What do you think will eventually happen?"**
  - **"Do you know anybody** who has had_____?" What was their life like?

Possible Goals (2)

- Treatment aimed at **cure** of the disease, including aggressive and experimental treatments
- Curative treatments but with **limited aggressive treatments**: no ventilator, no hospitalization, no feeding tube, and so on
- **Withdrawal** of selected or all of the current existing therapeutic interventions
- **Vigorous palliative care** with the **goal of quality of life** (i.e., maintaining functional capacity, pain control, comfort, and other symptom control)

Possible Questions to Ask

- "What makes you **happy**? How can we help you live as well as possible?"
- "Are there **special events or activities** that you are looking forward to?"
- "If you had to choose between quality of life and living longer, how would you **balance** this decision?"
- "What needs or services do you think you will need?"
- "How is your **family** involved?"
- "In what way do you think you could make your remaining time **meaningful?** How can we help?"

INVITE QUESTIONS FROM THE PATIENT

- Patients may want **time to reflect** on these issues.
- They may need to **hear the possible goals again** or **several times**.
- Agree on a **follow-up plan**.

SET THE GOALS

- Goals need to be **realistic**, but **don't take away hope** (see Chapter 16 on realistic hope).
- What specific **resources** will be needed to accomplish the goals?
- Remember that **goals usually change** throughout an illness: "I wanted to continue dialysis, but I'm just so weak that I don't want to go back anymore!"
- Reset **new goals** depending on where the patient is in the course of the disease.

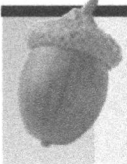

Goal Setting
IN A NUTSHELL

Goals should be discussed **early** in any serious illness.

"Cure" is only **one goal** out of many!

Once the patient's **goals are established, treatment decisions** become more **obvious.**

REFERENCES

1. Hammes BJ, Rooney BL. Death and end-of-life planning in one midwestern community. Arch Intern Med. 1998;158:383–390.
2. Crane MK, Wittink M, Doukas DJ. Respecting end-of-life treatment preferences. Am Fam Physician. 2005;72:1263–1268, 1270.

CHAPTER 21

The Hospice Conversation

Hospice provides a **unique range of benefits and services** for seriously ill patients. However, the decision to enroll in hospice is difficult and emotional. The public often equates "hospice" with "dying" and misunderstands that **hospice is about "living"** the best quality of life that is possible for as long as possible. It is the "quality" of life versus "quantity" of life decision, but emerging evidence suggests that many patients provided hospice/palliative care can actually have both (1).

THE PHILOSOPHY OF HOSPICE AND GOAL SETTING

Decisions in palliative care become easier once the patient's **goals** are known. As long as patients see death as an enemy and vow to "fight to the end," they are not ready to embrace death as a natural human event. But once the goals transition from "cure" to "palliation," hospice has much to offer:

- Patient's ability to die at **home** rather than in an institution
- Opportunity to remain in **control** of end-of-life decisions
- Chance to be surrounded by **loved ones and friends**
- A peaceful, pain-free, **natural death**

WHAT DOES HOSPICE PROVIDE?

Hospice is *not* "No care!" It is often **"more care."** Never say to a patient or their family, "There is nothing else we can do for you, so we are going to put you on hospice!"

> There may be nothing we can do to cure their disease, but there is always something we can do for the patient!

Hospice is paid for by the **Medicare Hospice Benefit**, Part A, and most insurance companies have a hospice benefit. Most hospices accept patients regardless of their ability to pay. The following are provided by most hospices:

- Home **nursing visits** (24-hour availability)
- **Social work** visits
- **Spiritual adviser** (usually a chaplain)
- **Home health aide** visits
- End-of-life **education** for the patient and family
- **Bereavement support** for 13 months after the death of the patient
- **Medications** related to the terminal diagnosis
- **Pain and symptom** management
- Durable **medical equipment** related to the terminal diagnosis
- Possibly incontinence supplies, wound care nurse visits, physician visits, nutritional support, and other benefits

WHO QUALIFIES FOR HOSPICE?

Entering hospice does not mean patients can never return to the hospital or change their mind at any time if they decide to pursue different treatments. Goals may change. Patients who qualify for hospice **generally have the following criteria**:

- The patient has chosen **palliation as a goal** rather than cure. However, DNR is *not* a prerequisite for hospice admission.
- There is an able and willing **caregiver** available. This does not have to be a family member; it can be the staff in long-term care. Some hospices have free-standing "hospice houses" that also provide these services.
- The patient chooses the **financial hospice benefit**—Medicare or other.
- There is a **terminal diagnosis**. In the past cancer was the prime hospice diagnosis. However now any life-limiting diagnosis is acceptable, including **end-stage cardiac disease, end-stage respiratory disease (COPD, pulmonary fibrosis, etc.), end-stage dementia, amyotrophic lateral sclerosis (ALS), end-stage renal disease, end-stage liver disease, and so on**.
- An average life expectancy of **6 months** or less. Because physicians are very poor at predicting life expectancy (2), the best question to ask is **"Would I be surprised if this patient died in the next 6 months?"**

> If there is any question about a patient qualifying, consultation with the hospice medical director is always appropriate.

THE 6-MONTH TEST

This is where most health care providers, as well as patients and families have difficulty. **No one can predict death with certainty**—otherwise we should be running life insurance companies!

Fortunately, CMS (Medicare) realizes that life expectancy is hard to predict. There is **no punishment if we predict wrong**! The **6-month test is a general one**.

- CMS (HCFA) states that the **physician does not need to know** if the specific individual will die in 6 months, but rather that individuals who present in the same way generally die in 6 months. (Medicare has not been explicit about the maximum expected survival rate at 6 months—for example, 10% or 50% survival!) (3)

- "The certification regarding terminal illness of an individual under paragraph (VII) shall be based on the physician's or medical director's clinical judgment regarding the normal course of the individuals illness" (4).

> **The better question is—"Would you be surprised if this patient died in six months?"**

DISCUSSING HOSPICE WITH THE PATIENT (5)

The discussion of hospice with a patient or the family should always be done in the context of **goals of care**. Ensure a comfortable setting with beepers and cell phones off, and then introduce the subject:

- "I'd like to talk to you about overall **goals** of your care."

- "What have the doctors told your?" Or, "What is your **understanding of this disease?**" If the patient does not understand his or her situation, then the hospice discussion may need to be delayed.

- "**What do you think** is going to happen in the future? What do you want to happen in the future?" **Listen carefully**.

- You may be able to **direct the conversation**—"What you are telling me is that you don't want to be a burden on your family, and you want to stay as independent as possible."

- Bring up the "H" word. "I know a lot of people don't understand what **hospice** is, but from what you are telling me, I think they can be very helpful in helping us achieve your goals." Explain that hospice is about **symptom management** and what is provided. Many people think you have to be actively dying to be on hospice or that it is a place people go to die. Answer questions **truthfully**. It's okay to say something like, "If you were my mother/brother/father, I would want hospice involved in your care!"

- Respond to **emotion**. Usually the emotional response is brief. Sitting quietly or a reassuring touch may help.

- **Offer a recommendation**—"From what we have talked about, I would recommend that someone from hospice come and talk to you."

- **Follow-up**. "After you have talked with the hospice people, I'll be back and we can talk more."

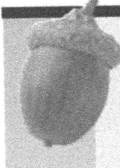

The Hospice Conversation
IN A NUTSHELL

Be familiar with the **philosophy of hospice** and the **benefits** that hospice can provide for the patient.

"Would you be **surprised** if this person died within the next 6 months?"

Approach the hospice discussion in context of **goals**.

Find out what the **patient understands** and what goals they have.

Repeat the goals back to the patient, and explain how hospice could help meet those goals.

Offer your **recommendation**.

Follow up.

REFERENCES

1. Cancer pain relief and palliative care. Report of a WHO Expert Committee. World Health Organ Tech Rep Ser 1990;804:1–75.
2. Christakis NA, Lamont EB. Extent and determinants of error in doctor's prognoses in terminally ill patients: prospective cohort study. BMJ. 2000;320:469–472.
3. Keay TJ, Schonwetter RS. Hospice care in the nursing home. Am Fam Physician. 1998;57:491–497.
4. Hospice care enhances dignity and peace as life nears its end. CMS Provider Education article. Available at: http://www.cms.hhs.gov/transmittals/downloads/ab03040.pdf. Accessed March 25, 2006.
5. Von Gunten C. Discussing hospice. *Fast Facts and Concepts*. National Residency End-of-Life Curriculum Project. Milwaukee: Medical College of Wisconsin; 2002.

CHAPTER 22

Telling the Children

Taking care of young adults who are dying is always hard but even more so when there are children in the family. However, if done correctly, health care providers have an opportunity to provide guidance to dying parents in preparing their children with adaptive coping skills that may affect them for the rest of their lives (1). There is great variability in children's grief reactions shaped by their developmental capacities (2).

AWARENESS

If the seriously ill person has children at home:

- Inquire about the children's ages, personalities, and any known coping skills.
- Find out what the children have been told about the parent's illness. Has there been a dialogue between the parent and the children?
- Ask if the child is having recent problems at school, at home, or with friends.

PREPARATION

Research supports the value of truthfully keeping the children informed about the parent's illness and the fact that he or she will die (3). Communication is key. The more painful a situation is for the adults, the more imperative it is to talk to the children about it. Children do not need every detail. What they critically need is an honest and convincing explanation (4).

Important things a parent can do in preparing the child for the parent's death include the following:

- Provide the children opportunities to ask questions and express their feelings.
- Express interest in the child's day.
- Try to maintain daily routines as much as possible. Special bonding times are great.

- Be honest and keep the child informed. The worse way to find out bad news is to overhear it.
- Involve the child. Let him or her express what they are thinking.
- Let the children know you love them, and that even though you will be going away, they are very important to you.
- Talk to the child's teacher or guidance counselor to let them know of the current situation at home.
- Physicians, social workers, and other health care providers can also meet with the children and provide support. Parents can be referred to one of several books on this subject.

THE DEATH

The family's response to the actual death of a parent depends on their culture, religious traditions, and ways of coping. Some families are able to handle caring for the patient at home with the help of hospice; others prefer terminal care in the hospital. Here are some ways of helping the child feel involved at the time of death:

- Visiting the dying parent in the hospital, although adolescents sometimes feel this is too emotionally painful. The medical team must balance the avoidance with making it clear that death is imminent and encouraging a final visit (1).
- Children may actualize the death by making pictures or picking out other keepsakes to bury with the parent in the casket.
- Encourage the surviving parent to allow the child to express grief through rituals, memorials, artwork, visiting the grave site, and so on.
- Children, as well as adults, may need to be relieved of irrational guilt.

BEREAVEMENT

Generally children and adolescents want to return to life as it was before the loss but recognize that life has forever changed. Therefore getting back to routine may be important. Successful reconstruction results in a decrease in the frequency and intensity of grief and sadness, although it never disappears.

The health care team should be vigilant for important symptoms of **abnormal grieving** that may require intervention:

- Regression in behavior beyond 6 months of the death
- Severe and persistent separation anxiety from the surviving parent for more than 6 months after the death
- Symptoms of significant depression that interfere with school, home, or friends
- Significant discord between the child and the surviving parent
- Risk-taking behavior
- Wanting to talk to someone outside the family

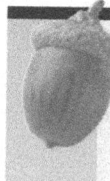

Telling the Children
IN A NUTSHELL

Screen for awareness: What are the ages of the children, and what do they know about the parent's disease?

Prepare the child: Communication is key. Children need honesty in the explanations that they receive.

Be honest to the children about imminent death. Encourage them to be present or to make a final visit. Defuse any feelings of irrational guilt that the child or adolescent may have.

Successful bereavement means getting back to a routine and the episodes of grief getting less intense and frequent.

Watch closely for symptoms of abnormal grief or prolonged grief lasting more than 6 months.

Refer if needed.

REFERENCES

1. Christ GH, Siegel K, Christ, AE. Adolescent grief—"It never really hit me . . . until it actually happened." JAMA. 2002;288:1269–1278.
2. Geis H, Whittlesey SW, McDonald NB, et al. Bereavement and loss in childhood. Child Adolesc Psychiatr Clin North Am. 1998;7:73–85.
3. Christ GH. *Healing Children's Grief: Surviving a Parent's Death from Cancer.* New York: Oxford University Press; 2000.
4. Keeley D. Telling children about a parent's cancer. BMJ. 2000;321:462–463.

CHAPTER 23

What If a Patient Asked You to Pray?

Health care providers are often seen as leaders or authority figures. As such, the frightened or distressed patient may ask them for prayer. How do we bring comfort and support to the patient without crossing the boundary of remaining true to our own beliefs? Furthermore, how do we prevent imposing our own values on a vulnerable patient?

OPTIONS

When patients request prayer, there are basically four options:

- **Pray with or for the patient**. If the caregiver sees that prayer will bring comfort to the patient, then it is hard to justify refusing, as long as health care providers feel confident in their own spirituality (1). One can only go as far with a patient on their spiritual journey as we have gone on our own.

  If the decision is made to pray with or for the patient, keep the prayer nondenominational or general. There are many different practices and beliefs. It is safest to ask for comfort or for God's will to be done, rather than specific outcomes.

- **Let the patient pray**. If caregivers are uncomfortable praying with or for a patient, they can choose to sit quietly while the patient prays. This way, they can add support to the patient's belief system without explicitly endorsing or influencing those beliefs (2).

- **Refer the request**. We are quick to refer in other areas of medical care but often don't entertain the idea of referring spiritual matters. Respectfully suggest that you would like to refer this request to an identified religious leader. This avoids the slightest suggestion of religious coercion on the caregiver's part (3). However, make that referral and make it quickly.

- **Respectfully decline**. Caregivers who are unprepared or uncomfortable with the preceding options may respectfully decline. However, it is important not to reject the patient. A truthful statement, such as "I'm sorry, but I am not really comfortable leading a prayer," is best. Other nonreligious supportive comments are also helpful, such as "You will be in my thoughts."

Important Points

- In all options, if a patient asks for prayer, it indicates **spiritual needs** and a professional chaplain or other spiritual leader should be consulted (4). See Chapter 14, "The Spiritual Assessment."

- Time is of the essence; don't delay or trivialize spiritual requests—they are very important to the patient.

- Do not say you are going to pray for a patient if you have no intention to do so. The lack of truth telling has the potential to undermine the healing relationship that you are trying to establish.

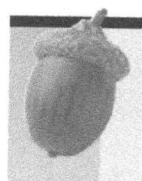

When Asked to Pray with Patients
IN A NUTSHELL

Pray if you are comfortable.

Sit quietly while the patient prays.

Refer to a spiritual leader.

Respectfully **decline**—but do not reject the patient.

Be truthful.

REFERENCES

1. Koenig HG. Religion, spirituality, and medicine: application to clinical practice. JAMA. 2000;284:1708.
2. Kwiatkowski KK, Arnold B, Barnard D. Physicians and prayer requests. *Fast Fact and Concept #120*, 2004. Available at: http://www.eperc.mcw.edu/FastFactPDF/Concept%20120.pdf. Accessed March 10, 2006.
3. Post SG, Puchalski CM, Larson DB. Physicians and patient spirituality: professional boundaries, competency, and ethics. Ann Intern Med. 2000;132:578–583.
4. Lo B, Ruston D, Kates LW, et al. Discussing religious and spiritual issues at the end of life: a practical guide for physicians. JAMA. 2002;287:749–754.

CHAPTER **24**

Death Pronouncement

"Please come and pronounce this patient!" Death is usually an **easy diagnosis** to make. Yet most health care providers get very little formal training on what to do (1,2).

BEFORE ENTERING THE ROOM

Certain information and **preparation** helps before entering the patient's room or home:

- Inquire about the **circumstances of the death**—expected or unexpected. If the death was outside a hospital, suspicious, or a child, the coroner may need to be called (this varies by state).
- Find out if the **attending physician** has been called. Most of the time in the hospital the patient can be pronounced and then the attending called.
- Is the **family present?** What is their condition—quietly grieving, dazed, angry, and so on?
- Has the family already talked to the **Organ Donor Network?**
- Are their special issues—**religious rituals or cultural requests?**
- Take a **deep breath** and **calm** yourself!

IN THE ROOM

Death pronouncement is a **solemn ritual**. Appear confident, calm, and professional at all times. Once in the presence of the patient:

- **Introduce yourself** to the family if they are present. Explain your relationship to the patient, and ask them their names and relationship to the patient.
- Tell the **family they are welcome to stay** if they wish. Some families prefer to leave while you examine their loved one.

THE PRONOUNCEMENT

Certifying death does not require any particular examinations (3). However, certain rituals are expected by the family:

- Note the **general appearance** of the body.
- **Identify the patient**—be sure it is who you think it is!
- Check for a **pulse**, radial or carotid—or both.
- Observe **breathing** motions—occasionally the clinician can be fooled by prolonged pauses such as in Cheyne-Stokes respirations.
- Auscultation of the heart/chest may be done.
- No further exam is needed. *Do not* do a **sternal rub**, nipple twisting, or other assessment for pain or shine a bright light into the pupils.
- **Record the time**.

> When entering the room, you can always buy time to think by taking the pulse while you decide what to do next!

TALK TO THE FAMILY

If the family is present, discuss the following:

- **Clearly communicate** that the person has **died**, and offer condolences.
- **Pause**—remain quiet and wait for their reaction.
- Answer **questions** that you can. If you can't, offer to find someone who can.
- Note if the family is requesting an **autopsy**.
- Find out which **funeral home** they wish to use.
- **Give permission** for the **family to spend some time** before they leave or before they enter into other decisions such as notifying other relatives.
- **Offer assistance** from clergy, a chaplain, or other religious leader as the family desires.
- When leaving the room, **model saying good-bye to the deceased**—a touch of the hand or forehead, or simply standing silent at the bedside for a few seconds.

DOCUMENTATION

Document the following in the patient's chart:

- "Called to pronounce (name)"
- "Patient found to be without pulse, respirations, or heartbeat [note other findings]."
- "Patient **pronounced dead at [date and time].**"
- Note if family was present or notified.

- Document if attending physician was notified and when.
- Document if family wants an autopsy.
- Document if the coroner was notified.

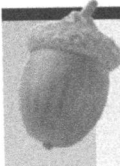

Death Pronouncement
IN A NUTSHELL

Prepare: What are the **circumstances** of the death? Is the **family present** and in what condition? Are there special **religious/cultural** requests?

Introduce yourself; get the names and relationships of family members. Let the family stay if they wish.

Pronounce: General observations. Pulse? Respirations? Heartbeat? A thorough examination is not needed. *Do not* do sternal rub, and so on. Record the time.

Talk to the family: State clearly that the person has **died**.

Offer **condolences**. Let the **family stay** if they wish. **Model** saying "good-bye" to the deceased.

Document: Be sure it's the **correct patient**; record the **date and time of death**; note if the family and attending were notified. Autopsy? Organ donation? Coroner?

REFERENCES

1. Weissman DE, Heidenreich CA. Death pronouncement in the hospital. *Fast Facts and Concepts # 4*. Milwaukee: The Medical College of Wisconsin; 2002.
2. Marchard LR, Kushner KP, Siewert L. Death pronouncement: survival tips for residents. Am Fam Physician, 1998. Available at: http://www.aafp.org/afp/980700ap/rsvoice.html. Accessed February 6, 2006.
3. Hallenbeck J. Palliative care in the final days of life—"they were expecting it any time." JAMA. 2005;293:2265–2271.

CHAPTER 25

Completing the Death Certificate

It is our **obligation** to our deceased patients and their families to complete the death certificate with the same professionalism and diligence that we showed in treating those patients during their lifetime. It is not rocket science. We merely need to be **timely, accurate, and specific** as to the cause of death.

IMPORTANCE OF THE DEATH CERTIFICATE

Besides the obvious importance of a death certificate, such as **proving death** before cremation or burial, it also has other far-reaching effects. Legally it is used in settling life **insurance claims, proving cancer policy claims, settling estates, closing bank accounts, selling stocks, deciding pension benefits, and providing evidence in court,** to name a few. Death certificates are also used as a primary tool in **measuring mortality rates and statistics** for grant funding and research. Therefore, the information reported on the death certificate often sets national, regional, state, and local priorities for **funding and research** (1).

MECHANICS OF SIGNING

Families and other agencies depend on the death certificate being legible and clearly reproducible by photocopy and microfilm. Use only permanent **black ink**. Correction fluid and erasures are not permitted. Avoid abbreviations.

Generally the funeral home will fill out everything except the physician's or medical part of the certificate. The certifier usually needs to enter the time of death.

WHO SIGNS THE DEATH CERTIFICATE

Ideally the physician who knows the most about the patient's cause of death signs the certificate. This may be the attending but could also be the consultant or the palliative care physician. These physicians may sign only for "natural" deaths (usually listed as "manner of death" on the death certificate). The coroner must sign for all unattended deaths, suspicious circumstances, homicides or suicides, accidents or trauma, and in most states the deaths of all children (2).

THE CAUSE OF DEATH

This is where thinking is involved. **Do not** enter the universal terminal event, such as **cardiac arrest or respiratory arrest**. Everyone's heart stops when they die, so that doesn't help much in statistics! Enter the **direct disease process that caused the death** (3). Ask yourself, "What disease process killed this patient?" Or, "Without what pathological process would this patient still be alive?"

In most cases, a time-linked **chain of causation** can be established. List the "immediate" cause of death, and then fill in the "Due to or As a consequence of" blanks. Other significant but not directly linked conditions are listed separately (4).

It is acceptable to list a **probable** diagnosis as long as it is reasonable. An example would be listing a metastatic carcinoma of unknown primary. "Unknown" should not be listed. If the cause of death is unknown, it is a case for the coroner!

If an **autopsy** is being performed, indicate **"pending"** and amend the certificate at a later date.

Examples:

1. Manner of death: Natural. Cause of death: Staphylococcal sepsis, due to methicillin-resistant staphylococcal pneumonia, due to chronic aspiration, due to Parkinson's disease.

2. Manner of death: Natural. Cause of death: Ventricular fibrillation, due to acute myocardial infarction, due to coronary artery thrombosis.

> No job is complete until the paperwork is done!

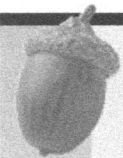

Completing the Death Certificate
IN A NUTSHELL

Be **timely**: Do not delay because the disposition of the body may be affected.

Write **legibly** and accurately.

Determine the "Manner of Death." If it is not **"natural,"** refer to the coroner or medical examiner's office.

Complete the **"Cause of death"** based on the disease process without which the patient would still be alive. Do not list universal terminal events such as "Cardiac arrest."

Complete the **"Due to**, or As a consequence of" section in logical order.

List **other significant diagnoses** separately.

Sign it.

REFERENCES

1. Swain GR, Ward GK, Hartlaub PP. Death certificates: let's get it right. Am Fam Physician. 2005;71:652.
2. Nowels D. Completing and signing the death certificate. Am Fam Physician. 2004;70: 1813–1818.
3. U.S. Department of Health and Human Services, Centers for Disease Control and Prevention. National Center for Health Statistics. Writing cause-of-death statements. 2004. Available at: http://www.cdc.gov/nchs/about/major/dvs/handbk.htm. Accessed March 5, 2006.
4. U.S. Department of Health and Human Services, Public Health Service, National Center for Health Statistics. Physicians' handbook on medical certification of death. Hyattsville, Md: U.S. Government Printing Office; 2003. DHHS publication no. PHS 2003–1108.

CHAPTER 26

Informing Significant Others of a Patient's Death

The public looks to the health care professional for information, reassurance, and direction when death occurs. Research shows that the sensitivity provided to family members regarding the **manner in which they receive word** that their loved one had died has a **lasting effect**. These memories and impressions may **affect the grief process** and the integration of the loss into the survivor's world (1).

Much of this information is contained in the chapters, **"Delivering Bad News," "Death Pronouncement,"** and **"Writing a Condolence Letter."** It is specifically organized here for convenience to use when informing significant others about a patient's death.

PREPARATION

- Examine the patient to **confirm death** (see Chapter 24).
- Find a **private place to meet** with the family. As a practical matter, this may be at the bedside of the deceased.
- If possible, learn the **names and relationships** of those you are talking with.

MEETING WITH THE FAMILY/SIGNIFICANT OTHERS

These skills of communication and compassion should be incorporated into the death notification process. Of course these will vary depending on the individual circumstances and whether or not the death was anticipated (2).

- **Introduce yourself** and find out **who is present**.
- **Respect** all religious, cultural, and ethnic traditions.
- Use **body language**—introductory handshake/hand clasp, eye contact, or touch that seems appropriate to the situation.
- Express your **sympathy**: "I'm sorry, but he/she is gone."

- Talk openly about the death—use **"died"** or **"dead"** during the initial conversation. Use the deceased name.

> Listen for key words used by the family to refer to death. For example, they may say "She passed" or "He died."

- Be prepared for **emotion**. Offering to order a mild sedative for a brief period of time to assist with insomnia is acceptable.

- **Answer questions**. Use nonmedical terms and reassure the family that the patient was comfortable, if it is true. Don't be afraid to say **"I don't know!"** Give information in layers, like "peeling an onion." Give one layer, and then proceed to the next if it is requested. Most of us tend to give too much information at a time when the mourners are not all that receptive.

- Offer **assistance** from other resources—chaplain, minister, social worker, and so on.

- Model **touching and saying good-bye** to the deceased (see Chapter 24).

- Offer the family some **alone time** with the deceased if desired.

- Offer to follow up and answer further questions.

FOLLOW-UP

- Personalize and send a **sympathy card or condolence letter** (see Chapter 27).

- Consider attending the **wake, funeral, or memorial service**. It is not inappropriate or unprofessional to grieve with the family!

- Continue **bereavement support**—watch for complicated grieving (see Grief: Uncomplicated vs. Complicated, Chapter 41).

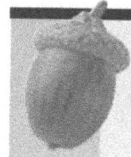

Informing Significant Others of a Patient's Death
IN A NUTSHELL

Prepare by **confirming death**, finding a **private place** to talk, introducing yourself, and finding out **who is present**.

Respect all traditions and culture.

Use **body language**.

Express **sympathy**.

Talk openly about the **death**: "Joe is dead."

Be prepared for **emotion**.

Answer questions.

Offer to **call** the chaplain, and so on.

Model saying good-bye to the deceased.

Follow up.

REFERENCES

1. Midland D. Informing significant others of a patient's death. *Fast Facts and Concepts # 64.* Milwaukee: Medical College of Wisconsin; 2002.
2. Hallenbeck J. Palliative care in the final days of life—"they were expecting it any time." JAMA. 2005;293:2265–2271.

CHAPTER 27

Writing a Condolence Letter

A letter of **condolence**, a **telephone call**, or a brief **visit** by the health professional shortly after the death of a patient is usually **welcomed** by the survivors. Writing a proper letter of condolence can contribute to the healing of the bereaved family (1).

WHY WRITE A LETTER OF CONDOLENCE?

Usually the reluctance on the part of the physician or other health care providers to approach the deceased patient's survivors stems from their perception that the family may be angry with them that the patient died. Many physicians see death as failure.

Good evidence, however, indicates that **bereavement outcomes** can be significantly **influenced by communication** and the quality of information and concern given to the patient's family. Providers who contact the bereaved survivors and express genuine concern and sorrow often minimize the anger that might otherwise be directed toward them (2).

Writing a letter of condolence also gives those who work in end-of-life care an **opportunity for** their own **closure**. Maintaining contact with the survivors for a short while after the loss of our patient often lets us see the courage, strength, love, and caring that their families exhibit during loss—and it gives us strength to continue our work in this area.

WHAT TO SAY

A good condolence letter has two main **goals**: to **offer tribute** to the deceased and to be a source of **comfort** to the mourners (3). These are the specific characteristics of a good condolence letter:

- Timely—written within **2 weeks** of the death.
- **Handwritten**—standard stationery or a card.
- Acknowledge the loss and name the deceased. Tell the bereaved how you learned of the death and how you felt on hearing the news. Using the **deceased's name** is a tribute that comforts most mourners.

- Express **sympathy**—"I'm sorry he/she's gone."
- Describe a **special quality** that you remember about the deceased. Mourners are always remembering the one who died, so don't be afraid to bring up memories. **Humorous stories** are especially appreciated by the bereaved.
- Pay tribute—"It was an **honor to know**_____!" "I will miss seeing him/her."
- Remind the **mourners** of their **special strengths**—"Joe was very lucky to have such a supportive family during his illness." Bereavement often brings self-doubt and anxiety. By reminding the survivors of their qualities (patience, optimism, faithfulness, etc.), it may help them cope.
- If an offer to help is made, **mean it**, and do it!
- End with a word or phrase of **sympathy**. Some phrases just don't make it, like "Sincerely" or "Fondly yours!" Try something like this: "You are in my thoughts and prayers," or "Remembering you and your family."

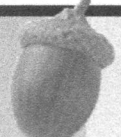

Writing a Condolence Letter
IN A NUTSHELL

Goals: Offer a **tribute** to the deceased and **comfort** to the bereaved.

Send the letter within 2 **weeks**.

It should be **handwritten**.

Acknowledge the loss; Use the **deceased's name**.

Express **sympathy**.

Describe a **special quality** of deceased or a memory that you have.

"It was an **honor** to know him/her."

Mention special attributes of the survivors.

Don't offer anything unless you mean it!

"You are in my thoughts and prayers!"

REFERENCES

1. Bedell SE, Cadenhead K, Graboys TB. The doctor's letter of condolence. National Vital Statistics Reports Final Data, 1998. N Engl J Med. 2001;344:1161–1162.
2. Main J. Improving management of bereavement in general practice based on a survey of recently bereaved subjects in a single general practice. Br J Gen Pract. 2000;50:863–866.
3. Wolfson R, Menkin E. Writing a condolence letter. *Fast Facts and Concepts*. Milwaukee: Medical College of Wisconsin; 2002.

CHAPTER 28

Caring for the Family

Each patient is a member of a family unit that has its own unique characteristics, communication styles, and individual needs. When we meet the patient and family in palliative care, they are often in crisis. It is important that our plan of care (POC) includes input from the palliative care (PC) team, patient, and family to thoroughly address the supportive and educational needs of the seriously ill and/or dying patient.

> Definition of family: the biological relatives and those people identified by the patient as significant.

Assessment Skills

- Maximize listening skills.
- Minimize quick judgment.
- Be sensitive to patient/family readiness to discuss end-of-life issues and to identify new goals of care (1,2).

> "Listen or your tongue will make you deaf."

Family Assessment

- Check the family's understanding of the diagnosis and prognosis: "What are you expecting to happen and when?"
- Identify the decision maker and primary caregiver.
- Identify concurrent issues such as: recent loss, multiple losses, financial concerns, prolonged illness, or problems coping.
- Is the family system supportive, enmeshed, estranged, disconnected, or other?
- Identify primary language and cultural traditions regarding illness and death.
- Are there changes in family members' roles and responsibilities?

- Assess for the so-called elephant-in-the-room issues, such as alcohol/drug abuse or broken relationships.
- Identify parents' needs about informing the children, and assess the coping of children by asking about their fears/concerns.
- Identify what the patient/family value and how the patient and family describe quality of life (QOL) for the patient.
- Does the patient have an advanced directive or AND/DNR status?
- What are the spiritual needs or concerns?
- Has the family considered funeral plan and preferences of the patient as appropriate?
- Identify educational needs.

> "Happiness is having a large, loving, caring, close-knit family—in another city." —George Burns

Intervention

- Normalize the patient's and family's experience.
- Assist the family in identifying coping strategies.
- Provide education about the illness trajectory, symptom management rationale, and signs of impending death when appropriate.
- Provide information about hospice and other community support services.
- As appropriate to the family dynamics, help patient and family complete the "Five Things That Matter Most" (3):
  - Please forgive me.
  - I forgive you.
  - Thank you.
  - I love you.
  - Good-bye.
- Encourage the family to tell stories of their life together

> *Telling our family's story:* "In the hearing is the learning; in the telling is the healing."—C. Scanlon, RN

Important Needs of the Family

- To be with the person and to feel helpful.
- To be informed of changes in condition in a timely manner.
- To understand what is being done and why.
- To be assured of the patient's comfort.
- To be comforted and know that we care.
- To be able to vent emotions in a safe environment.

- To be assured that their decisions on behalf of the patient are appropriate.
- To find meaning in the patient's illness and death.

> "It is OK to say that everyone wishes it had turned out differently."—Karin Porter-Williamson, MD

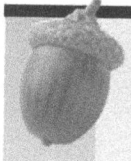

Caring for the Family
IN A NUTSHELL

Trust building

Education

Listening—letting the steam blow off

Scheduling family meetings

Providing care and attention to the family, which gives comfort to the patient

REFERENCES

1. King DA, Quill T. Working with families in palliative care: one size does not fit all. J Palliat Med. 2006;9:704–715.
2. Rolland JS. Mastering family challenges in illness and disability. In: Walsh F, ed. *Normal Family Processes*. 3rd ed. New York: Guilford; 2003:460–489.
3. Byock I. The four things that matter most: A book about living. New York: Free Press; 2004.

Predicting Life Expectancy

CHAPTER 29

"How Long Do I Have?"

Determining life expectancy during the course of terminal illness is difficult. But one of the most common questions asked by individuals at the end of life is, *"How long do I have?"* **It is best to answer this question in general rather than specific terms.** Use phrases such as:

- Months to years
- Weeks to months
- Days to weeks
- Hours to days

Weeks to Months
- Increased discomfort
- Decreased appetite
- Increased fatigue and sleep
- Talk about dying
- Decreased ability to perform activities of daily living (ADLs)

Days to Weeks
- Very poor oral intake
- Nausea
- Rapid or labored respirations
- Excess pulmonary or gastric secretions
- Decreased alertness but responsive
- Decreased blood pressure
- Increased pulse
- Decreased urinary output

Hours to Days

- Inability to walk (if previously able)
- Diaphoresis
- Poor thermoregulation
- Dreams or visions of deceased loved ones
- Disorientation
- Agitation
- Picking at clothes or the air

CHAPTER 30

Guidelines for Hospice

Medicare coverage of **hospice care** depends on a physician's certification of an individual's prognosis of a **life expectancy of 6 months or less if the terminal illness runs its normal course.**

Why refer patients to hospice?

- Allows patients to remain at home until the end of their life.
- Offers team-based approach to meet physical, emotional, and spiritual needs of the patient and also their caregivers.
- Provides medical equipment and medications related to terminal illness.
- Improves patient and family satisfaction with health care at the end of life.

When to Refer Patients to Hospice

- Patient meets 6-month prognosis criteria.
- Patient and family choose palliative care instead of curative care.
- Patient is not currently receiving therapy under Medicare Part A for the same diagnosis as the hospice diagnosis.

What Is Attending Physician's Role with Hospice?

- Provide initial certification of terminal illness and order for hospice services.
- Continue to provide patient's health care management including direct hands-on care or diagnostic interpretation services.
- Provide input and update of patient's plan of care by consulting with hospice.

HOSPICE FACTS

Hospice Benefits

- Specialized services of **pain management**
- **Psychosocial and spiritual care**

- **Medical equipment**
- **Medications** related to the terminal illness
- **Bereavement support** for family for at least 1 year

Levels of Care

- **Routine home care**
- **Respite care** in a Medicare-approved long-term care facility or hospital for up to 5 consecutive days
- **Inpatient care** in a Medicare-approved long-term care facility or hospital
- **Continuous care** for up to 24 hours per day at the patient's bedside during times of crisis management

Myth Busters

- Hospice patients can continue to receive medical care from their attending physician for all illnesses *related and unrelated* to their terminal condition.
- Hospice patients may receive the following Medicare benefits for conditions *unrelated* to their terminal condition:
  - Hospitalization
  - Skilled care benefits in a long-term care facility
  - Home health services
  - Medical care from physicians other than the hospice and attending physician
- Hospice patients are not required to have a DNR.
- Hospice provides the same services to patients in a long-term care facility as in any other home setting.

CHAPTER 31

Physician Prediction of Life Expectancy

Because of physician optimism in evaluating terminal illness, patients are typically referred to hospice late in the course of illness, resulting in underutilization of hospice benefits. The median length of stay in hospice is less than 3 weeks, and many patients receive hospice care for only several days (1,2).

Hospice Services

- In-home care

- Expertise in pain and symptom management

- Services for caregivers

Introducing information about hospice early in the course of illness facilitates informed decision making regarding life-sustaining treatments versus palliative care. Late referrals to hospice limit access to the services that hospice offers (2).

In determining prognosis for hospice appropriateness, the question physicians should be asking themselves is, *"Would I be surprised if this patient died within the next 6 months?"*

Several indicators are helpful in predicting the life expectancy of a terminally ill patient. Clinical factors include a decline in functional status in these areas:

- Cognitive functioning
- ADLs
- Incontinence and nutrition
- Weight loss
- Increase in falls
- Changing hematology values

Nonclinical factors that indicate possible nearing of the end of life include the following:

- Mood and personality change
- Social withdrawal
- Loneliness

REFERENCES

1. Casarett DJ, Crowley RL, Hirschman KB. How should clinicians describe hospice to patients and families? J Am Geriatr Soc. 2004;52:1923–1928.
2. Oliver DP, Porock D, Zweig S. End-of-life care in U.S. nursing homes: a review of the evidence. J Am Med Dir Assoc. May/June 2004:147–155.

CHAPTER 32

Palliative Performance Score

The Palliative Performance Scale (PPS) is a modification of the Karnofsky Performance Scale. **The Palliative Performance score is useful in predicting poor survival. It takes into account ambulation, activity, self-care, intake, and conscious level.** A score of **50% or less** may indicate a prognosis of 6 months or less (see Table 4). **Cancer patients** who are determined to be hospice appropriate by their attending physician are **not required to meet any other clinical guidelines**.

TABLE 4

Palliative Performance Scale

%	Ambulation	of disease	Self-Care	Intake	Level
	Activity & Evidence		**Conscious**		
100	Full	Normal activity/no	Full	Normal	Full evidence of disease
90	Full	Normal activity/ some	Full	Normal	Full evidence of disease
80	Full	Normal activity with effort/some evidence of disease	Full	Normal or reduced	Full
70	Reduced	No normal job/work/ some evidence of disease	Full	Normal or reduced	Full
60	Reduced	No hobby/housework significant disease	Occasional assistance needed	Normal or reduced	Full or confusion
50	Mainly sit/lie	Unable to do any work extensive disease	Considerable assistance needed	Normal or reduced	Full or confusion
40	Mainly in bed	As above	Mainly assistance	Normal or reduced	Full or drowsy or confusion

(continued)

TABLE 4 (Continued)

Palliative Performance Scale

	Activity & Evidence			Conscious	
%	Ambulation	of disease	Self-Care	Intake	Level
30	Totally	As above	Total care	Reduced bedbound	Full or drowsy or confusion
20	As above	As above	Total care	Minimal sips	Full or drowsy or confusion
10	As above	As above	Total care	Mouth care only	Drowsy or coma
0	Death	——	——	——	——

CHAPTER 33

Specific Diseases:
Noncancer Diagnoses

Recognizing that determining life expectancy during the course of a terminal illness is difficult, the Centers for Medicare & Medicaid Services (CMS) has established medical **criteria for determining prognosis** for **noncancer diagnoses**. *The patient may not meet all of the criteria, yet still be appropriate for hospice care because of other co-morbidities or a rapid decline.*

CONGESTIVE HEART FAILURE

1 and 2 must be present:

1. Patient is already optimally treated with diuretics and vasodilators, or has a medical contraindication for those drugs, or has made a conscious decision not to take them.

2. Patient has significant symptoms of recurrent congestive heart failure (CHF) at rest (i.e., inability to carry on any physical activity without discomfort; and if any physical activity is undertaken, discomfort is increased). Significant CHF may be documented by an ejection fraction of <20% but is not required if not already available.

   Factors that will add supporting documentation:

- Symptomatic arrhythmias
- History of cardiac arrest or resuscitation
- History of unexplained syncope
- Brain embolism of cardiac origin
- Concomitant HIV disease
- Angina pectoris, at rest
- History of previous myocardial infarction

CHRONIC OBSTRUCTIVE PULMONARY DISEASE

*1 must be present with either 2 **or** 3:*

1. Severe chronic lung disease as shown by *both a and b*:
    a. Disabling dyspnea at rest, poorly or unresponsive to bronchodilators, resulting in decreased functional capacity (e.g., bed-to-chair existence, fatigue, and cough). (Documentation of forced expiratory volume in 1 second [FEV_1], after bronchodilator, <30% of predicted is objective evidence for disabling dyspnea, but it is not necessary to obtain.)
    b. Progression of end-stage pulmonary disease, as evidenced by increasing visits to the emergency department or hospitalizations for pulmonary infections and/or respiratory failure. (Documentation of serial decrease of FEV_1 <40 mL per year is objective evidence for disease progression, but it is not necessary to obtain.)
2. Hypoxemia at rest on room air, as evidenced by Po_2 <55 mmHg and oxygen saturation <88% on supplemental oxygen *or* hypercapnia, as evidenced by Pco_2 <50 mmHg.
3. Cor pulmonale and right heart failure (RHF) secondary to pulmonary disease.

   Factors that will add supporting documentation:

- Unintentional progressive weight loss of greater than 10% of body weight over the preceding 6 months.
- Resting tachycardia >100 beats per minute.

AMYOTROPHIC LATERAL SCLEROSIS

Any one of these clinical findings demonstrating a rapid progression of ALS must be present within 12 months preceding initial hospice certification:

1. Progression from independent ambulation to wheelchair or to bed-bound status
2. Progression from normal to barely intelligible or unintelligible speech
3. Progression from normal to pureed diet
4. Progression from independence in most or all activities of daily living to needing major assistance by caretaker

   In addition, any of the following constellation of clinical problems will signify terminal illness:

1. Critically impaired breathing capacity

    Vital capacity (VC) <30% of normal

    Significant dyspnea at rest

    Requiring supplemental oxygen at rest

    Patient declines invasive artificial ventilation

2. Critical nutritional impairment

    Oral intake of nutrients and fluids insufficient to sustain life

    Continuing weight loss

    Dehydration or hypovolemia

    Absence of artificial feeding methods

3. Life-threatening complications

    Recurrent aspiration pneumonia

    Upper urinary tract infection (e.g., pyelonephritis)

    Sepsis

    Fever recurrent after antibiotic therapy

    Decubitus ulcers, multiple, stage 3–4

DEMENTIA

At least four of the following criteria must be present:

1. Unable to ambulate without assistance
2. Unable to dress without assistance
3. Unable to bathe without assistance
4. Urinary and fecal incontinence, intermittent or constant
5. No meaningful verbal communication: stereotypical phrases only or the ability to speak is limited to six or fewer intelligible words

   *Must have had one of the following **or some other documented significant condition** in the past 12 months*:

- Aspiration pneumonia
- Pyelonephritis or other urinary tract infection
- Septicemia
- Decubitus ulcers, multiple, stage 3–4
- Fever, recurrent after antibiotics
- Inability to maintain sufficient fluid and calorie intake with 10% weight loss during the previous 6 months or serum albumin <2.5 g per dL

LIVER DISEASE

1 and 2 must be present:

1. The patient should show *both a and b*:

    a. Prothrombin time (PT) >5 seconds over control *or* international normalized ratio (INR) >1.5

    b. Serum albumin <2.5 g per dL

2. End-stage liver disease is present and the patient shows *at least one* of the following:

    a. Ascites

    b. Spontaneous bacterial peritonitis

    c. Hepatorenal syndrome: elevated blood urea nitrogen/creatinine (BUN/CR), oliguria

    d. Hepatic encephalopathy

    e. Recurrent variceal bleeding

Factors that will add supporting documentation:

- Progressive malnutrition
- Muscle wasting with reduced strength and endurance
- Continued active alcoholism (>80 g of ethanol per day)
- Hepatocellular carcinoma
- HBsAg (Hepatitis B) positivity
- Hepatitis C refractory to interferon treatment

Patients awaiting liver transplant who otherwise fit the preceding criteria may be certified for the Medicare hospice benefit, but if a donor organ is procured, the patient must be discharged from hospice.

RENAL DISEASE

1, 2, and 3 must be present:

1. The patient is not seeking dialysis or renal transplant.
2. Creatinine clearance <10 mL per minute (<15 mL per minute for diabetics)
3. Serum creatinine >8.0 mg per dL (>6.0 mg per dL for diabetics)

*Factors lending supporting evidence for **acute** renal failure*:

- Mechanical ventilation
- Malignancy (other organ system)
- Intractable hyperkalemia (>7.0)
- Uremic pericarditis
- Hepatorenal syndrome
- Intractable fluid overload
- Immunosuppression/AIDS
- Albumin <3.5 g per dL
- Cachexia

- Platelet count <25,000
- Disseminated intravascular coagulation
- Gastrointestinal bleeding
- Chronic lung disease
- Advanced cardiac disease
- Advanced liver disease
- Sepsis

*Factors lending supporting evidence for **chronic** renal failure*:

- Uremia
- Oliguria (<400 mL per day)
- Intractable hyperkalemia
- Uremic pericarditis
- Hepatorenal syndrome
- Intractable fluid overload

CEREBRAL VASCULAR DISEASE

Acute phase of hemorrhagic or ischemic stroke
*1, 2, **or** 3 must be present*:

1. Coma or persistent vegetative state beyond 3 days
2. In postanoxic stroke, coma or severe obtundation accompanied by severe myoclonus beyond 3 days
3. Dysphagia that prevents sufficient intake of foods and fluids to sustain life and no artificial nutrition/hydration

Chronic phase of hemorrhagic or ischemic stroke
*1, 2, **or** 3 must be present*:

1. Poststroke dementia *(all of the following)*

    Unable to ambulate without assistance

    Unable to dress without assistance

    Unable to bathe without assistance

    Urinary and fecal incontinence, intermittent or constant

    Ability to speak six or fewer intelligible words
2. Poor functional status with Palliative Performance Scale score 40% or less
3. Poor nutritional status with >10% weight loss during the previous 6 months or serum albumin <2.5 g per dL

AIDS

1 and 2 must be present:

1. CD4+ count <25 cells/mc/L or persistent viral load >100,000 copies per mL, *plus one* of the following:

   CNS lymphoma

   Wasting (loss of 33% lean body mass)

   Mycobacterium avium complex bacteremia

   Progressive multifocal leukoencephalopathy

   Systemic lymphoma

   Visceral Kaposi sarcoma

   Renal failure in the absence of dialysis

   Cryptosporidium infection

   Toxoplasmosis

   Advanced AIDS dementia complex

2. Decreased performance status, as measured by the Palliative Performance Status scale, of 50% or less.

   Factors that will add supporting documentation:

- Chronic persistent diarrhea for 1 year
- Persistent serum albumin <2.5 g per dL
- Concomitant, active substance abuse
- Age >50 years
- Absence of antiretroviral, chemotherapeutic, and prophylactic drug therapy
- Toxoplasmosis
- Congestive heart failure, symptomatic at rest

GENERAL DEBILITY

No specific number of criteria must be met.
They are listed in the order of their power to predict poor survival.

1. Progression of disease as documented by symptoms, signs, and test results
2. Decline in Palliative Performance Scale score
3. Weight loss
4. Dependence on assistance for *two or more* activities of daily living:

   Feeding

   Ambulation

   Continence

  Transfer

  Bathing

  Dressing

5. Dysphagia leading to inadequate nutritional intake

6. Decline in systolic blood pressure or progressive postural hypotension

7. Increasing need for skilled service

8. Decline in cognitive function

9. Progressive stage 3–4 pressure ulcers in spite of optimal care

OTHERS

*The patient should meet **all** of the following criteria:*

1. Life-limiting condition

2. Patient/family informed condition is life limiting

3. Patient/family elected palliative care

*plus **one or more** of these criteria:*

4. Documentation of clinical progression of disease

  Evidenced by one or more of the following:

- Laboratory studies
- Radiologic or other studies
- Multiple emergency department visits
- Inpatient hospitalizations
- Home health nursing assessment if patient homebound

and/or

5. Recent decline in functional status

  Evidenced by either:

- Palliative Performance score of 50% or less

 or

- Dependence in three or more activities of daily living

and/or

6. Recent impaired nutritional status

  Evidenced by either:

- Unintentional, progressive weight loss of 10% over past 6 months

 or

- Serum albumin <2.5 g per dL

REFERENCES

1. *Medicare Reference Guide for Hospice Agencies, Coverage Guidelines*, September 2003.
2. Palmetto GBA. *Medicare Part A Hospice Training Manual*, 2005.

Delivery of Palliative Care

CHAPTER 34

The Hospital Palliative Care Unit

Aging demographics, human suffering, compassion, and economics are pushing hospitals toward palliative care (1). As with any new paradigm of health care, the process is still evolving, but current trends include some or all of the following characteristics:

- **In-patient consultation service**: Usually an interdisciplinary team made up of physicians, midlevel practitioners, social workers, chaplains, an ethics committee, wound care specialists, and others. This group serves to educate others about palliative care.

- A **palliative care ward or room**: Used much like a "hospice house" but doesn't require moving the patient. It is available at a much lesser charge than a bed in the intensive care unit, for example.

- A **palliative care philosophy**: Hospitals with formal palliative care availability are shown to have **better patient and caregiver satisfaction** ratings, **improved pain and symptom control, shorter length of stay** (streamlined care), and **lower hospital costs** (2). (Palliative care does not make money, but it saves money!) The **integration of palliative with curative models earlier** in the course of life-threatening illness is also well recognized (3).

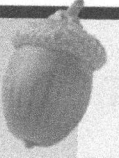

The Hospital Palliative Care Unit
IN A NUTSHELL

Integrating palliative care with traditional curative models is still **evolving** in the hospital setting.

Hospitals providing palliative care are reporting **superior patient satisfaction, improved pain and symptom control,** and **lower hospital costs.**

It is the **right** thing to do!

REFERENCES

1. Fine RL. The imperative for hospital-based palliative care: patient, institutional, and societal benefits. Proc (Baylor Univ Med Cent). 2004;17:259–264.
2. Morrison RS. Health care system factors affecting end-of-life care. J Palliat Med. 2005; 8(suppl 1):S79–S87.
3. Passik SD, Ruggles C, Brown G, et al. Is there a model for demonstrating a beneficial financial impact of initiating a palliative care program by an existing hospice program? Palliat Support Care. 2004;4:419–423.

CHAPTER 35

Consulting in the Hospital

Special nature of palliative care consultation: "It's not just another consult . . ."

WHAT DO WE DO?

- **Mediation** of many providers' thoughts regarding patient history, condition, treatment options with attendant risks and benefits, and prognosis, all to arrive at a "consensus opinion" from the medical perspective.

- **Integration** of that consensus opinion into the patient and family's worldview, to arrive at a treatment plan focused on patient- and family-specific goals of care.

- **Action plan initiation**: Whole person assessment and interdisciplinary management of patient and family needs through course of illness.

- **Resolution**: The plan of care plays out, either to stabilization and disposition from the hospital or not, with end-of-life care taking place in the hospital or other end-of-life care setting.

WHAT MAKES PALLIATIVE CARE CONSULTATION SPECIAL?

- High stakes in plan of care for patient and family.

- Oftentimes big decisions are at hand.

- Discussion and recognition of serious illness and life change has a ripple effect through many families' foundations: Hardiness of family structure is tested, and strengths and weaknesses in coping styles are revealed.

- Shift in paradigm to patient-centered rather than disease-focused care. It's not just another day in the neighborhood, so to speak, and people know they are being approached differently by their system of care.

- High stakes for the medical providers:
  - We all need to know we've done our best.
  - We all need to feel safe knowing that death is not our personal failure.
  - We all need support in posing the question "whose needs are the plan of care serving: the patient's, the family's, mine?"

CONSULTANT'S ROLE: HOW DO WE APPROACH OUR ROLE AS CONSULTANT?

Pure consultation model: Consultant offers specific recommendations and expertise regarding a problem while the primary attending physician explicitly maintains locus of control, making all final management decisions.

Co-management model: Consultant manages specific problems, writing orders as necessary, while the primary attending physician continues to guide overall plan of care.

Assumption of care model: Consultant assumes the locus of control for patient's plan of care and all specific management decisions.

Consult Etiquette

Know your clients—who are they?

Attending physician

Other physicians, nurses, and ancillaries caring for patient

There are usually many people involved in the patient's care, all with relevant input for you about how the patient is doing and what the patient is feeling. Capitalize on their knowledge and elicit their opinion. It will come out somewhere, so it's best to put it all on the table.

THE "DO" LIST

1. **Communicate with the primary attending *always* and *first*.** Here are some questions to ask:
   - "How can I help you with this situation? Are there particular concerns that you want to make sure we are aware of?"
   - "What are your goals for this patient/What are you hoping will happen?"
   - "In your opinion, what is likely to happen?"

2. If there is something about the patient's current plan of care that you don't understand or agree with, ask about it in a nonthreatening way (e.g., "Help me to understand what we (not *you*) are hoping to achieve by doing X . . .").

3. Advocate your position ahead of time: "On my review of the situation, what stands out to me are A, B, and C. Would you tend to agree with me?" "After discussion with the patient and family, they may choose to do X, Y, or Z. Are you comfortable with these potential outcomes?

4. Commiserate with them and tell them it's obvious how much they care, if that seems true to you. They probably wouldn't be calling if it was a happy story with a great ending. They need your support too.

5. **Make the expectations regarding locus of control explicit**. Ask, "Would you like me to leave recommendations only, or would you like me to write orders as I feel appropriate?" This is a show of respect for the physician as the attending. Over time you will come to know how different physicians prefer to handle the situation.

6. Some physicians are explicitly uncomfortable with end-of-life situations. Rescue them to the extent they wish to be rescued. Offer to take the patient if you feel this will best serve the patient and family needs.

KNOW YOUR STUFF

In discussions with patient and family, know what all of the providers think about the situation so a uniform message is communicated. Tell the other providers what you are communicating so everyone is on the same page! In your treatment recommendations, know what best practice is and advocate for it.

BE RESPONSIVE

They are calling because they perceive a need. If you shut them down and say it's not important, they may not call again.

FOLLOWTHROUGH

Act in the manner of consultation agreed on, and follow up on the symptoms, the psychosocial issues, the spiritual needs, and the necessary goals discussions, no matter how many, to solidify a plan of care that makes sense to the patient, family, and care providers.

THE "DON'T DO" LIST

1. **Don't demean your client and call them names if they've engaged in a ridiculous plan of care for months on end**. You won't get invited back the next time.

2. You weren't there the whole time to see how decisions got made along the way—no Monday morning quarterbacking!

3. **Don't demean your client in front of patient or family**. It's unprofessional.

4. The patient and family need to know that all of their care providers are on their side, not fighting with one another about who is right or wrong.

5. **Don't demean your client in the patient record**. If the medical professionals disagree, this should spawn an interdisciplinary conference to hash it out. No chart wars!

6. **Don't say "no" to your clients** without offering an alternative or compromise strategy for getting them help with whatever their problem is (e.g., pain management consult).

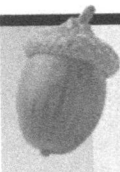

Consulting in the Hospital
IN A NUTSHELL

Palliative care consultation always holds high stakes. No other specialists enter the scene under such emotional circumstances.

Communication is key—with the patient, family, staff, and attending physicians.

CHAPTER 36

Hospice in Delivery of Palliative Care

Hospice is currently the primary method of delivering palliative care in the United States (1). Originally a renegade alternative medicine option, hospice has rapidly become the standard of care for terminal patients. Medicare pays for about 80% of all hospice care (2).

WHAT HOSPICE PROVIDES

The number of hospice programs continues to increase in the United States, from 1 program in 1974 to 2,312 in 1994 and 3,650 in 2004 (1). All hospice companies and organizations must, by Medicare standards, provide minimum services including the following:

- Case oversight by a physician
- Nursing visits—24/7 emergency availability
- Social work visits
- Home health aides
- Spiritual care—usually a chaplain
- Volunteer services
- Bereavement support to the family after the death
- Medications consistent with the terminal diagnosis
- Durable medical equipment (hospital bed, commode, wheelchair, etc.)
- Other services: Some hospice organizations provide wound care, incontinence supplies, speech therapy, physical therapy, occupational therapy, nutrition support, and so on.

ELIGIBILITY: MEDICARE HOSPICE BENEFIT

- Patient must be entitled to Medicare Part A (hospital benefits). They must sign off of the hospital benefit and onto the hospice benefit, but this can be reversed at any time.

- Patient must be certified by the hospice medical director and one other physician, usually the attending if there is one.
- DNR status cannot be used as a requirement.

DIAGNOSIS

Patients are certified to have a life expectancy of less than 6 months *if* the disease runs its natural course (which is unusual!). Patients continue to qualify after the initial 6-month certification period if the medical director believes death is likely within the next 6 months. These are the most common diagnoses:

- Cancers
- End-stage heart disease/congestive heart failure (CHF)
- Dementia
- Debility
- End-stage pulmonary disease
- End-stage renal disease
- Amyotrophic lateral sclerosis (ALS)
- End-stage Parkinson's disease
- Cerebrovascular accident (CVA)
- Other terminal illnesses

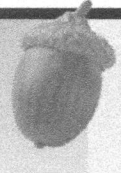

Hospice in Delivery of Palliative Care
IN A NUTSHELL

Hospice provides most of the outpatient palliative care.

There are specific Medicare guidelines for hospice organizations.

Any terminal diagnosis qualifies a patient for hospice services.

REFERENCES

1. National Hospice and Palliative Care Organization statistics. Available at: www.nhpco .org/nds.
2. Centers for Medicare & Medicaid Services. Hospice Center. Available at: http://www.cms .hhs.gov/center/hospice.asp. Accessed July 9, 2006.

CHAPTER 37

Hospice in the Nursing Home

Hospice services are being used more frequently in the long-term care setting. More than 25% of Americans now die in a nursing home, and considerable evidence indicates that residents of long-term care do not receive optimal end-of-life care (1). The interdisciplinary support of the **hospice team** can be **invaluable** in **supporting the usual nursing home care** at a time when staff, family members, and the patient are facing the increased and urgent needs associated with the dying process (2).

BENEFITS OF HOSPICE IN LONG-TERM CARE

Many health care providers, patients, and patients' families are becoming aware that a **goal of comfort** is more satisfying and reasonable for patients in long-term care than aggressive life-prolonging goals (3). The Medicare hospice benefit can make it much easier for nursing home staff, physicians, and other providers to give comprehensive palliative care to terminally ill patients.

Good evidence indicates that nursing home residents who receive hospice services are more likely to have **good pain assessment** and management, have **lower rates of inappropriate medication usage**, and are less likely to have **physical restraints** (4).

Here are some other **advantages** of involving hospice in the care of the terminally ill patient in the nursing home:

- Terminally ill patients can be kept in their **own environment**, and the natural dying process can be respected. Most dying patients prefer to remain in their usual setting.
- Specially trained hospice professionals (physicians, nurses, social workers, chaplains, etc.) and volunteers can provide many services that are beyond those usually offered in long-term care.
- The medical **goal** becomes pain relief and symptom control.
- Terminal patients' increasing **hygienic needs** are managed.
- Hospice provides end-of-life **education** for the family and for the nursing home personnel.

- Hospice offers **bereavement support** for the family and for the nursing home staff, who often become emotionally close to the patients.
- **Prolonged visits** can provide compassionate listening and companionship.
- **Medications** and **medical supplies** related to the terminal diagnosis are available.
- **Spiritual support** is offered.
- **Hospitalizations** and life-prolonging therapies are limited.
- Surviving family members report greater **satisfaction** with the nursing home.
- There is **education by osmosis** to the nursing home staff on end-of-life care when hospice professionals are on site.

BARRIERS TO HOSPICE IN LONG-TERM CARE

Federal policy emphasizes **rehabilitation and restoration** of function as the goals of nursing home care. Reimbursement is tied to this focus. Yet, at the end of life, all indicators of successful restoration are going to fail. Add to this the fact that nursing homes are the most heavily regulated industry in the United States. Many survey domains, such as weight loss, anorexia, functional decline, and increased usage of opioids and antipsychotic medication, are common in palliative care. Therefore, **goal setting** and **documentation** become imperative to avoid this "clash of philosophies."

Here are some other common barriers to high-quality end-of-life care in long-term care facilities:

- Many long-term care facilities **do not have established procedures** for ensuring that patients receive hospice services (5).
- Most patients in long-term care have multiple co-morbidities, including progressive dementia in more than half. This makes **life expectancy estimates much more difficult**. These patients are more likely to be referred later than patients with a cancer diagnosis, which is much more predictable (6).
- High staff turnover in long-term care is typical.
- Staff training is limited and there is insufficient staffing (7).

OVERCOMING THE BARRIERS

Although hospice might not be the right choice for all terminal patients in long-term care, good evidence indicates that measurable **outcomes are improved when hospice is involved**. Methods to overcome the barriers to that care include the following:

- **Communication** between patients, physicians, families, nursing home staff, hospice professionals, and others
- **Support** for advanced care planning
- Goal setting
- Proper **documentation**—by the hospice as well as by the long-term care facility
- Appropriate **earlier referrals** to hospice
- **Education**

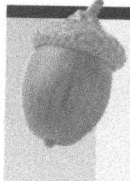

Hospice in the Nursing Home
IN A NUTSHELL

Good evidence indicates that **supplemental hospice services** (in addition to usual services) in the terminally ill patient in the nursing home improve medical outcomes as well as family and patient satisfaction.

Barriers to hospice in the nursing home include emphasis on restoration, lack of communication, and difficulty in predicting life expectancy in this population.

Communication, goal setting, documentation, and education can overcome the barriers.

REFERENCES

1. Casarett D, Karlawish J, Morales K, et al. Improving the use of hospice services in nursing homes. JAMA. 2005;294:211–217.
2. Keay TJ, Schonwetter RS. Hospice care in the nursing home. Am Fam Physician. 1998;57:491–497.
3. The care of dying patients: a position statement from the American Geriatrics Society. J Am Geriatr Soc. 1995;43:577–578.
4. Miller SC, Mor V, Teno J. Hospice enrollment and pain assessment and management in nursing homes. J Pain Symptom Manage. 2003;26:791–799.
5. Petrisek AC, Mor V. Hospice in nursing homes: a facility-level analysis of the distribution of hospice beneficiaries. Gerontologist. 1999;39:279–290.
6. Zerzan J, Stearns S, Hanson L. Access to palliative care and hospice in nursing homes. JAMA. 2000;284:2489–2494.
7. Hanson LC, Ersek M. Meeting palliative care needs in post-acute care settings "To help them live until they die." JAMA. 2006;295:681–686.

Terminal Care

CHAPTER 38

The Syndrome of Imminent Death

When patients are allowed to die naturally, the body begins to shut down and the **syndrome of imminent death** (actively dying stage) can be recognized (1). It is important for both the clinician and the family to be aware of and to be prepared for this situation. Key factors are described next.

Early Stage

- Bedbound
- Loss of interest in eating or drinking
- Increased sleepiness
- Near-death awareness/delirium

Midstage

- Fever common
- Further decline in mental status—often obtunded
- So-called death rattle: pooling of oral secretions because of the loss of the swallowing reflex

Late Stage

- Cool extremities/mottling
- Coma—unresponsive to painful stimuli
- Fever common—often from aspiration pneumonia
- Altered respiratory pattern—either fast or slow, with periods of apnea common
- Death

CONSIDERATIONS

The **time course** to traverse these stages is **difficult to predict accurately**. It can vary from less than **24 hours** up to **10 to 14 days** (2). Family can be told that we are now talking in "days" and not "weeks" or "months."

Food and **water** are **unnecessary** at this stage because the body is shutting down. Family members should be informed of this, as they often feel their loved one is hungry or thirsty. The patient is dying from a disease, not from lack of nutrition (3).

TREATMENT FOR IMMINENT DEATH SYNDROME

Symptoms often escalate as death approaches, and even families that are well informed may begin to question their ability to handle the situation (4). Just the availability of an experienced clinician is tremendously comforting. The following are important measures:

- **Keep the family informed**. Explain that the patient is actively dying. **Document "patient is dying,"** not "prognosis is poor or guarded."

- Discuss **stopping all treatments** that are not contributing to comfort—fingersticks, oral medications, intravenous (IV) lines, antibiotics, and so on.

- **Death rattle**: Use **scopolamine patches**—one or two (two is the palliative care dose, but you must write "for palliative treatment" on the prescription or the pharmacy may not fill it!). May also use **atropine eye drops** orally 2 to 4 drops titrated every 4 hours as needed or in patients with an IV, **glycopyrrolate, 0.4 to 0.8 mg** may be given every 4 to 8 hours as needed.

- Titrate morphine drops (Roxanol, 20 mg per mL) to control **dyspnea** or **tachypnea**. The goal should be to keep the respiratory rate in the range of 10 to 15.

- **Continue opioids to treat pain**. Do not stop pain medications as death approaches. Assume the pain stimulus is still present; families like reassurance that their loved one is not suffering.

- Provide **mouth and skin care**.

- Let the family know that just **being present** is the most important thing they can do for their loved ones at this stage.

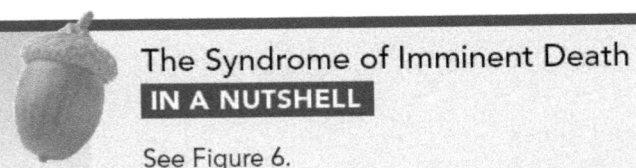

The Syndrome of Imminent Death
IN A NUTSHELL

See Figure 6.

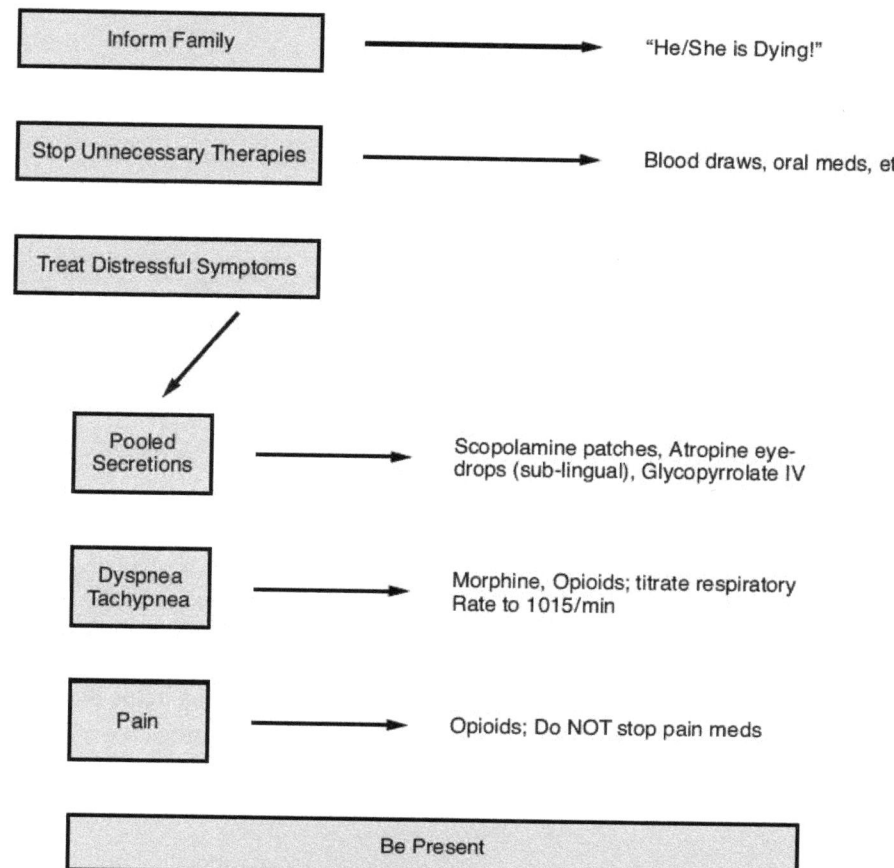

FIGURE 6 ● The Syndrome of Imminent Death

REFERENCES

1. Weissman DE. Syndrome of imminent death. *Fast Fact and Concept #3*. 2nd ed. July 2005. End-of-Life Palliative Education Resource Center. Available at: http://www.eperc.mcw.edu/fastFact/ff_003.htm. Accessed June 25, 2006.
2. Furst CJ, Doyle D. The terminal phase. In: Doyle D, Hanks G, Cherny NI, et al., eds. *Oxford Textbook of Palliative Medicine*. 3rd ed. New York: Oxford University Press; 2004: 1117–1133.
3. McCue JD. The naturalness of dying. JAMA. 1995;273:1039–1043.
4. Taylor GJ, Kurent JE. *A Clinician's Guide to Palliative Care*. Malden, Mass: Blackwell; 2003.

CHAPTER 39

Near Death Awareness

Near death awareness (NDA) is a widely reported phenomenon that many people experience during the dying process (1). Information on this topic is anecdotal and can be **misinterpreted as delirium**. Caregivers, family, friends, and health professionals must be **aware of NDA** and not react with fear, frustration, inappropriate medication, or annoyance, which just causes further isolation and suffering for the dying patient.

Delirium presents with **deficits** in orientation, short-term memory, or attention. **NDA**, in contrast, is a **positive phenomenon** that is often **comforting to the patient**. Like in dreams, the language patients use to communicate NDA may be **symbolic** and hard to understand.

With patience and active listening, health professionals, family, friends, and caretakers can help decipher NDA messages (2).

WHAT NDA LOOKS LIKE

Patients may appear confused or disoriented, or as if they are dreaming. The difference between NDA and delirium may be difficult. Recognition of NDA requires attentive listening. These experiences can be very comforting for patients but often unsettling to observers. Common phenomena include the following:

- Speaking to people who others cannot see.
- Reaching out as though trying to touch someone who can't be seen.
- Gesturing, waving, or holding an unseen object.
- Describing "angels," bright colors, light, or a peaceful place.

Two broad categories of messages are described:

Attempts to Describe What Dying Is Like

- Experiencing the presence of, or communicating with dead relatives, friends, or others
- Describing a place that they see in another realm

- Preparing for travel or a significant change
- Predicting when their death will occur
- Describing a feeling of peacefulness

Final Requests for a Peaceful Death

- Need for closure or forgiveness in a personal or spiritual relationship
- Closure on some ethical matter
- Removing some barrier to a peaceful death
- Preparing for death via specific items or rituals

Unlike delirium, NDA is not uncomfortable to the patient and does not generally need medical intervention.

PEARLS FOR DEALING WITH NDA PHENOMENA

Medication is generally not needed for NDA. The person who is emotionally closest to the patient may best understand what is being said (3). The following measures apply:

- Accept and validate what the patient is telling you; do not argue or challenge. These experiences can be very comforting to the patient.
- Evaluate for causes of delirium if the patient seems uncomfortable; treat when appropriate.
- Be present. Sit at the bedside and be open to a patient's attempts to communicate.
- Be aware that agitation may be arising from a message not being understood or addressed.
- Gently ask the patient about messages you don't understand. "Who or what do you see?"
- Be honest when you don't understand, but let the patient know you will keep trying.
- Be honest about patients' approaching death and that they may be experiencing things we don't understand.
- Help the patient find closure if specific issues are involved: If issues can be identified, specific people may be able to address them (relative, friend, chaplain, rabbi, priest, etc.).
- If you don't know what to say, be silent but be present.
- Provide education and support about NDA to others who are present. This event may have a powerful impact on the lives of others (4).
- Lessen your own fears about dying.

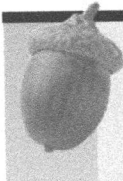

Near Death Awareness
IN A NUTSHELL

Be aware that NDA exists; it is not dangerous to the patient.

Educate caregivers, family, friends, and others about NDA.

Accept and validate what the patient is telling you—**don't argue.**

Listen attentively—fix the things you can fix.

Help the patient find closure.

Be present—just being there may be better than words.

REFERENCES

1. Marchard L. Near death awareness. *Fast Fact and Concept #118*. Available at: http://www.eperc.mcw.edu/fastFact/ff_118.htm. Accessed March 25, 2006.
2. Callahan M, Kelley P. *Final Gifts:Understanding the Special Awareness, Needs and Communications of the Dying.* New York: Simon & Schuster; 1992.
3. The Hospice of the Flordia Suncoast. Nearing death awareness. Available at: http://www.thehospice.org/deathaware.htm. Accessed March 25, 2006.
4. Kircher PM, Callanan M. Near-death experiences and nearing death awareness in the terminally ill. International Association for Near-Death Studies; 2003. Available at: http://www.iands.org/terminally_ill.html. Accessed February 19, 2006.

CHAPTER 40

Terminal Delirium

Most patients experience some degree of cognitive loss or confusion in the week or two before death (1). The cause is often hard to identify and may be related to multiple factors.

PRESENTATION

Delirium presents as either one of two ways:

- **Agitated/hyperactive delirium**: climbing out of bed, pulling out IV, picking at air, wild behaviors, incoherent speech
- **Hypoactive-hypoalert delirium**: quiet, very sleepy, hard to arouse, mumbling speech

DIFFERENTIAL DIAGNOSIS

Causes of terminal delirium are multiple—at least 40% of the time they are never determined. However, common causes include the following (1,2):

- **Metabolic**: hypoxia, hypercalcemia, hyponatremia, hypoglycemia, liver or renal failure, dehydration
- **Central nervous system (CNS) pathology**: metastases, infarction, ischemia, bleeding, infection
- **Drug withdrawal**: alcohol, benzodiazepines, barbiturates
- **Drug toxicity**: benzodiazepines, opioids, steroids, illicit drugs, alcohol
- **Other**: systemic infections, fever, heart failure, imminent death, urinary retention or constipation, sleep deprivation

ASSESSMENT

- Perform an examination—look for easily reversible common causes: drug effects, hypoxia, fever, hypotension, sleep deprivation, and so on.

- Distinguish between delirium and dementia:
  - *Dementia* refers to a chronic loss of intellectual function with diminished memory, thinking, and judgment.
  - *Delirium* is an acute confusional state that often includes hallucinations and perceptional disturbances.
- Determine if the patient is in danger of harming themselves or others. Is this state distressing to the patient? (Note: Near death awareness (see Chapter 39) is often comforting to the patient!)
- If clinically appropriate and desired by the caregivers, labs can be done to search for a treatable cause. However, most of the time in palliative care, this is not practical.

TREATMENT

Ideal treatment includes identifying and treating the cause of the delirium.

Nondrug Therapy

- Provide a quiet, well-lit room; a night light may help.
- Placing the patient next to a window may help.
- Ask a family member or health professional to be present for support—or to leave if they seem to upset the patient!
- Avoid physical restraints. These usually make the situation worse!
- Rehydration may be helpful to correct dehydration or to dilute metabolic or drug toxicity.

Drug therapy is indicated for patients who are a danger to themselves or others, distressfully agitated, or are severely sleep deprived. The most useful drugs include neuroleptics; however, benzodiazepines are still used (3).

Drug Therapy

- **Neuroleptics: First Line**
  - Haloperidol (Haldol): Start with 1 to 2 mg PO, IV, IM, or SC every 2 hours as needed, and titrate upward (4).
  - Chlorpromazine (Thorazine): 12.5 to 50 mg PO, IV, IM, or SC every 6 hours, and titrate upward 25 mg every hour as needed.
- **Atypical neuroleptics**: May be helpful, but evidence is still pending, so they are not considered first line (5).
  - Olanzapine (Zyprexa): 5 mg PO every day for 1 week; then 10 mg every day; may be titrated to 20 mg per day.
  - Quetiapine (Seroquel): 25 mg PO twice daily; may be increased 25 to 50 mg per dose every 2 to 3 days to 300 to 400 mg per day, divided into two to three doses.
  - Risperidone (Risperdal): 1 to 2 mg PO at night and increased 1 mg every 2 to 3 days to 4 to 6 mg PO at bedtime.

- **Benzodiazepines**: Can cause a **paradoxical reaction** with **increasing agitation**. These are no longer recommended for delirium. Too many clinicians reach for the Ativan first! Try haloperidol!

- If **opioids** are needed for pain, they should be **continued**, but the **dose** can be adjusted if appropriate.

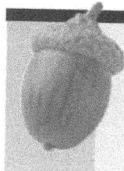

Terminal Delirium
IN A NUTSHELL

Terminal delirium is an acute confusional state that is common in patients nearing death.

Appropriate assessment should be done, but the causes are often multifactorial.

Terminal delirium may not need treatment unless it is dangerous or distressful to the patient.

Nondrug treatments include reorientation, leaving a light on, providing a window, and having people present.

Haloperidol (Haldol) is the drug of choice. Titrate 1 to 2 mg every hour to effect (maximum, 10 mg); then 1 to 2 mg every 6 hours.

Benzodiazepines may cause a paradoxical reaction.

REFERENCES

1. Weissman DE, Ambuel B. *Improving End-of-Life Care: A Resource Guide for Physician Education.* 2nd ed. Milwaukee: Medical College of Wisconsin; 1999.
2. Ingham JM. Delirium. In: Berger A, Portenoy R, Weissman DE, eds. *Principles and Practice of Supportive Oncology.* Philadelphia: Lippincott-Raven; 1998.
3. Brietbart W, Marotta R, Platt M, et al. A double blind trial of haloperidol, chlorpromazine and lorazepam in the treatment of delirium. Am J Psych. 1996;153:231–237.
4. Weissman DE. Diagnosis and management of terminal delirium. *Fast Facts and Concept #1.* 2nd ed. July 2005. Available at: www.eperc.mcw.edu. Accessed July 14, 2006.
5. Pharmacologic management of delirium; update on newer agents. *Fast Facts and Concepts #60*; Quijada E, Billings, JA, eds. January 2002. Available at: www.eperc.mcw.edu. Accessed July 14, 2006.

CHAPTER 41

Grief: Uncomplicated vs. Complicated

Loss through death is extremely stressful. In dealing with end-of-life patients, our job is not done until we are assured that those close to our patient are grieving appropriately. No one else is in a better position to observe and distinguish between normal and pathological grief reactions in the family and friends of our patient. Empathic aftercare for bereaved patients demonstrates our respect for the deceased and concern for the surviving family members. Growing evidence indicates that the aftercare of those caring for the deceased patient can make a positive difference in the grieving process of those remaining (1).

UNCOMPLICATED GRIEF

Grief is not a disease that can be cured. It is a normal process related to significant loss. Normal, or uncomplicated, grief reactions are those that, although painful, move the survivor toward an acceptance of the loss and an ability to carry on with his or her life (2). Indicators of normal adjustment include many of the following:

- Accepting the loss as real and the life changes that are unavoidable.
- Capacity to feel that life still has meaning.
- A continued sense of self-efficacy—taking care of one's health, eating right, and so on (avoiding harmful behaviors).
- Ability to trust in others—engaging in social pursuits.
- The capacity to reinvest in interpersonal relationships and activities (e.g., being involved with family and making new friends).
- Although always painful, thoughts of the loss of the deceased occupy less of one's thoughts with the passage of time.

COMPLICATED OR "PATHOLOGICAL" GRIEF

Some persons are at high risk for complicated grief, and they deserve enhanced attention following a significant loss:

- Who was lost: The more dependent the relationship, the greater the risk for complicated grief. The loss of a child is very high risk.

- How the loss occurred: Sudden, unexpected, and untimely deaths increase risk of complicated grieving; especially suicides, homicides, mutilations, and so on.

- Personal history: Poor coping abilities in the past, history of psychiatric illness (depression, anxiety, etc.), history of substance abuse.

- Social factors: Frequent geographical moves, separation from support groups, estrangement and lack of cultural norms or role models for grieving.

- Simultaneous stressors: Multiple losses, economic problems, job changes or loss, recent geographical moves, legal problems, and so on.

Everyone has a unique way of grieving. To complicate matters, grief does not progress in an orderly fashion through various stages on a timeline (3). However, several red flags can be indicators of complicated or pathological grieving:

- Patient is unable to accept the loss (disbelief or searching for the deceased) and make changes in response to the new situation.

- Severe grief that is stuck and not changing or improving over 6 months to 1 year.

- Delayed grief: The loss has initially overwhelmed the person's ability to cope. People seem to be doing "too well" at first, but minor events trigger intense reactions even years after the death.

- Severe isolation: withdrawal, loss of job, and so on.

- Excessive irritability, bitterness, or anger.

- Risk-taking behaviors including abuse of alcohol and prescription drugs.

- Avoidance of self-care and health matters, including nutrition.

- Frequent physical complaints.

- Depression and/or anxiety.

MANAGING COMPLICATED GRIEF

Grieving is normal with any significant loss. Therefore quick attempts to prevent the pain of loss with medication are usually not helpful. When patients and families are allowed to feel the deep pain of loss, they are more likely to approach healing (4).

The following interventions may be helpful in treating complicated grief:

- Rule out physical disease, including medical depression.

- Listen: Bereaved patients want to talk about heir loss. Do not avoid talking about the deceased, even if it is painful—it may help get appropriate grieving back on track.

- Provide education to normalize the grieving process.

- Validate the pain and help the patient express it.

- Provide ongoing support from a skilled interdisciplinary team such as hospice.
- Refer to mental health professionals if needed.
- Assess for suicidal ideation and take appropriate measures.

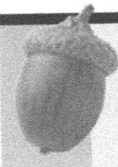

Uncomplicated vs Complicated Grief
IN A NUTSHELL

In normal grieving:

Loss is accepted.

Pain is not gone but gets better with time.

Life continues to have meaning.

There is avoidance of harmful behaviors.

Social contacts continue.

In complicated "pathological" grieving:

Inability to accept the loss.

Grief is static—does not progress with time (6–12 months).

Delayed grief: Minor events trigger intense feelings.

Social withdrawal.

Excessive anger or irritability.

Risk-taking behaviors—alcohol/drugs.

Poor self-care.

REFERENCES

1. Main J. Improving management of bereavement in general practice based on a survey of recently bereaved subjects in a single general practice. Br J Gen Pract. 2000;50:863–866.
2. Prigerson HG, Jacobs SC. Caring for bereaved patients—"All the doctors just suddenly go." JAMA. 2001;286:1369–1376.
3. Parkes CM, Weiss R. *Recovery from Bereavement.* New York: Basic Books; 1983.
4. Storey P, Knight CF. Alleviating psychological and spiritual pain in the terminally ill. UNIPAC Two, *Hospice/Palliative Care Training for Physicians.* 2nd ed. Glenview, Illinois: American Academy of Hospice and Palliative Medicine; 2003: 51.

Nonpain
Symptom
Management

CHAPTER 42

Tips for Maximizing Chances of Success

- Maximize patient and family control.

- Try to anticipate and prevent symptoms.

- If you educate patients/families before symptoms (e.g., dry mouth, Cheyne-Stokes breathing) occur, they will be grateful.

- Elicit help from interdisciplinary team.

- Note that risk of failure is increased by:

  - Cognitive impairment

  - Minority status (e.g., being African American) (1)

  - Language barrier

See Figure 7 for a list of symptoms (2).

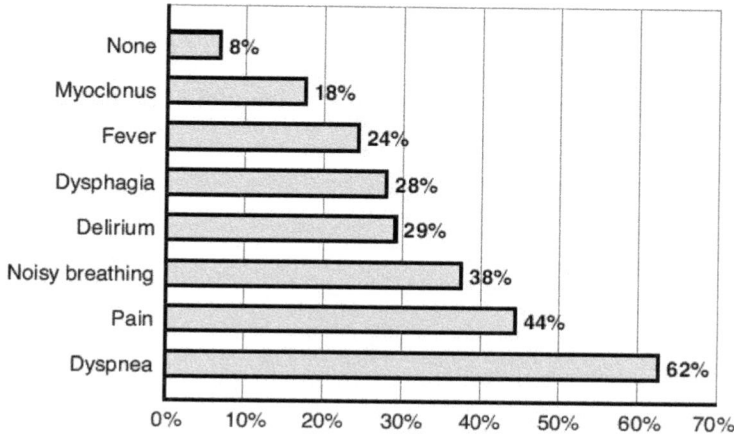

FIGURE 7 ● Symptoms in dying long-term care patients, 1999 Ottawa Chart Review

REFERENCES

1. Krakauer EL, Crenner C, Fox K. Barriers to optimum end-of-life care for minority patients. J Am Geriatr Soc. 2002;50:182–190.
2. Hall P, Schroder C, Weaver L. The last 48 hours of life in long-term care: a focused chart audit. J Am Geriatr Soc. 2002;50:501–506.

CHAPTER 43

Dyspnea, Air Hunger, Shortness of Air

General Considerations

- Common at all stages of dying
- *Subjective* sensation of uncomfortable breathing:
    - *Not* linked to measurements of blood gases, respiratory rate, or oxygen saturation
- May limit activity and quality of life
- Strongly associated with anxiety:
    - Each may cause or exacerbate the other
    - Very frightening to patient and caregivers

Common Causes of Dyspnea

- **Pneumonia**
- **Bronchospasm**
- **COPD**
- **Mucus plugs**
- **Pulmonary embolism**
- **Pleural effusion**
- **Fecal impaction, urinary retention**
- **Severe anemia**
- **CHF**
- **Cardiac ischemia**
- **Cardiac arrhythmia**
- **Tumor invasion**
- **Damage from radiation and chemotherapy**

Dyspnea Assessment and Management

- Symptom history and physical examination
- Workup based on benefits and burdens, patient's prognosis, preferences, goals
- Find what works for this person:
  - Positioning, fan (works via V2 branch of fifth cranial nerve), open window, relaxation techniques
  - *Trial* of oxygen (4 to 6 L per minute by nasal cannula) based on symptom relief
  - Avoid suctioning in most patients (can be distressing)

Opioids: Treatment of Choice for Dyspnea

- **Morphine is most studied and versatile**
- For opioid-naive patients:
  - Immediate-release morphine, 5 to 15 mg PO every 4 hours
  - Sustained-release morphine, 15 to 30 mg PO every 12 hours
  - Hydromorphone, 0.5 to 2 mg PO every 4 hours
  - Oxycodone, 5 to 10 mg every 4 hours
- For patients on opioids, increase up to 50%
- If dyspnea is intermittent, use as needed may be okay

Other Medications to Consider for Dyspnea

- **Benzodiazepines** for anxiety:
  - Lorazepam, PO/sl/IV, 0.5 to 1 mg PO every 4 hours
- **Bronchodilators** for wheezing
- **Chlorpromazine** (Thorazine):
  - 10 to 25 mg every 4 to 6 hours
  - May work synergistically with morphine
- Steroids, diuretics, anticoagulation, erythropoietin in appropriate settings

Treatment to Suppress Cough

- **Guaifenesin with dextromethorphan** (Robitussin DM):
  - Dextromethorphan related to codeine
- **Codeine, Hydrocodone**:
  - Beware of constipation!
- **Chlorpromazine** (Thorazine):
  - 25 mg PO/IM every 4 to 6 hours for cough triggered by hiccups

Anticholinergics to Dry Secretions

- **Anticholinergics' other potential benefits**:
  - Decrease gastrointestinal secretions and acidity, relax tracheobronchial smooth muscle
  - Useful in bowel obstruction (if octreotide, i.e., Sandostatin, not needed or not available)
- **Glycopyrrolate (Robinul)**:
  - 0.1 to 0.2 mg IM or 1 to 2 mg PO two or three times daily
  - Only agent not crossing blood–brain barrier, so treatment of choice in frail patients
- **Scopolamine, Atropine, Hyoscyamine (Levsin)**: All cross blood–brain barrier

CHAPTER 44

Oral Care Basics

General Considerations

- Frequent physician examination:
    - Especially to rule out infection (e.g., thrush)
- Oral care *at least* daily (if conscious):
    - At least three to four times daily if unconscious
- Wonderful way to involve family
- Detailed oral care routines:
    - University of Ottawa Institute of Palliative Care (www.pallcare.org/educate)

Oral Care Tips

- Effective mouthwashes:
    - Sodium bicarbonate (5 mL in 500 mL normal saline)
    - Plain club soda
- To help clean debris:
    - Fresh pineapple (ananase is proteolytic)
- For coated tongue:
    - Sucking on vitamin C tablets
    - 3% hydrogen peroxide with equal parts water (only if there are no open oral lesions; unpleasant taste, so rinse with plain water)

Dry Mouth

- Use whatever works:
    - Frequent sips of favorite liquids, popsicles, frozen fruit or fruit juices or tonic water, hard candies, artificial saliva
    - Avoid alcohol mouthwashes, glycerine swabs

- **If patient unconscious:**
    - Swab the mouth every 1 to 2 hours with water or normal saline.
    - Spray with an atomizer.
- **Vaseline to lips and front teeth**
- **Review anticholinergics**

CHAPTER 45

Fever Near the End of Life

General Considerations

- Discuss possible infections *ahead of time* as part of advance care planning.
- Onset may trigger a time of decision.
- Consider benefits and burdens of workup and treatment in light of:
  - Current stage of illness; prognosis
  - Patient's preferences and goals of care
- Fever itself usually responds to acetaminophen.
- Communication and documentation is needed.

CHAPTER 46

Agitation and Anxiety

General Considerations

- Keep an open mind during assessment:
    - Ask, "What's going on here?"
    - Try to make sense of the behavior rather than leaping to control measures (sedatives, restraints).
    - Talk (listen) to patient and family.
- May have physical *and* psychological causes:
    - For example, urinary retention, anxiety, *and* delirium
    - Often a sign of pain in cognitively impaired
- Environment may be a cause.
- Evaluation of symptoms will yield best clues.

Management

- Likely to require multifactorial interventions
- Environmental modification(s)
- Psychological support
- Medications:
    - Neuroleptics (for delirium)
    - Antidepressants
    - Benzodiazepines (for anxiety, not for delirium)
    - Morphine (for dyspnea, pain)

CHAPTER 47

Sexual Needs

General Considerations

- Sexual and intimacy needs continue beyond diagnosis of illness.
- Patient, family, and staff attitudes may hinder intimacy.
- Often patients and families need reminders and permission that intimacy is okay.
- Lying together may be deeply meaningful.
- Staff should attend to privacy and dignity.

CHAPTER 48

Spiritual and Existential Suffering

General Considerations

- Spiritual pain is common.
- Cultural more than religious differences affect how we experience suffering.
- Clinicians can play a powerful role in eliciting and acknowledging spiritual concerns:
  - Should not feel compelled to address them oneself
- Organizational interventions:
  - Pastoral counseling, volunteers, diverse scriptures and sacred objects, music

Suffering: Recognition Most Important Step

- *Suffering is individual.*
- "Making a diagnosis of suffering means first of all maintaining a high index of suspicion in the presence of serious disease and obviously distressing symptoms."
- "As a start, it means asking whether the patient is suffering and why."

CHAPTER 49

Nausea and Vomiting

Nausea

- Subjective sensation caused by stimulation of chemoreceptor trigger zone, cerebral cortex, vestibular apparatus, gastrointestinal lining (see Table 5)

Vomiting

- Neuromuscular reflex triggered in medulla (vomiting center)

See Figure 8 for pathophysiology of nausea/vomiting and Table 6 for common mechanisms and treatment.

Illustrative Nausea Treatments

- **Prochlorperazine (Compazine)**:
    - Potent antidopaminergic, weak antihistamine, anticholinergic agent
    - Preferred for opioid-related nausea
- **Haloperidol**:
    - Very potent antidopaminergic agent

TABLE 5

Origins of Nausea

• CTZ (via rising opioid levels)
  • The most common mechanism: 28% of patients
  • Transient (3–7 days) if dosing is steady.
  • Long-acting forms facilitate steady dosing.
	• Upper GI dysmotility (gastroparesis)
	  • Less common
	  • Tolerance does not develop
	• Vestibular apparatus
	  • Unusual; note spinning sensation
	• Constipation, impaction

CTZ, chemoreceptor trigger zone; GI, gastrointestinal.

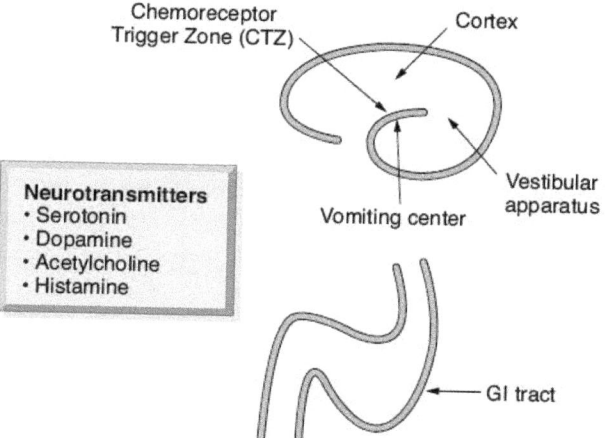

FIGURE 8 • Pathophysiology of Nausea/Vomiting

- **Promethazine (Phenergan):**
  - Antihistamine with potent anticholinergic properties, very weak antidopaminergic agent
  - Useful for vertigo and gastroenteritis caused by infections and inflammation
  - *Not* useful for opioid-related nausea
- **Scopolamine:**
  - A very potent, purely anticholinergic agent

Nonpharmacological Interventions for Nausea

- Cool damp cloth to forehead, neck, wrists
- Bland, cool, or room temperature foods

TABLE 6

Common Mechanisms and Treatment

Sites	Triggers	Treatments
Cortex	Learned behavior	Lorazepam
CTZ	Rising opioid levels	Prochlorperazine
	Digoxin	Haloperidol
	Metabolic (Na, Ca)	
Vestibular apparatus	Opioids (unusual)	Scopolamine
	ENT (usual)	Promethazine
GI irritation	NSAIDs, Fe	Promethazine
Upper GI dysmotility	Opioids	Metoclopramide
	Anticholinergics	
Lower GI obstruction	Constipation	Bowel measures
	Impaction	

Ca, calcium; CTZ, chemoreceptor trigger zone; ENT, ears, nose, and throat; Fe, iron; GI, gastrointestinal; Na, sodium; NSAIDs, nonsteroidal anti-inflammatory drugs.

- Decrease noxious stimuli (e.g., odors, noise)
- Limit fluids with food
- Fresh air, fan
- Relaxation techniques
- Acupuncture/pressure or transcutaneous electrical nerve stimulator (TENS) to P6:
  - Midline wrist, 3 cm from palmar crease
- Oral care after each emesis

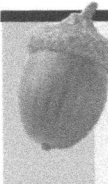

Nausea and Vomiting
IN A NUTSHELL

Origins of nausea and vomiting:

Cortex

CTZ (chemoreceptor trigger zone)

Vomiting center

Upper GI dysmotility (gastroparesis)

Vestibular apparatus

Constipation, impaction

Treatments for nausea and vomiting:

Lorazepam, 0.5 to 1 mg every 6 hours as needed

Prochlorperazine, 10 mg every 4 to 6 hours as needed

Haloperidol, 0.5 to 1 mg every 4 to 6 hours as needed

Scopolamine, 1 to 3 patches every 3 days

Promethazine, 12.5 to 25 mg every 4 to 6 hours as needed

Metoclopramide, 10 mg three to four times daily before meals

ABHR (Ativan, Benadryl, Haldol, Reglan) gel, 1 mL every 4 to 6 hours
    as needed, or suppository, 1 PR every 4 to 6 hours as needed

Bowel measures

Nonpharmacological interventions for nausea and vomiting:

Cool cloth

Bland, room temperature foods

Decrease stimuli

Limit fluids with food

Fan

Relaxation

Acupuncture or acupressure

Dizziness

Vertigo

- Medications: Review medication list for etiology:
    - Amitriptyline (Elavil)
    - Metoclopramide (Reglan)
- Treatment:
    - Meclizine (Antivert), 12.5 to 25 mg three times daily
    - Scopolamine (transdermal patch), every 72 hours

Syncope

- Micturition syncope: Avoid sitting
- Postural hypotension
- Reduce or discontinue diuretics and antihypertensives
- Discontinue amitriptyline or metoclopramide
- Discontinue sodium restriction
- Oral rehydration
- If anemic, consider blood transfusion

Transient Ischemic Attack (TIA)

- ASA (aspirin), 50 to 325 mg every day
- Discontinue and avoid warfarin (Coumadin) and heparin because of increased risk of bleeding

Teaching for Caregivers

- Advise the patient to move slowly.
- Avoid swift head movements.
- Avoid looking upward.

- Avoid postural hypotension:
    - Lying position to sitting position
    - Sitting position to standing position

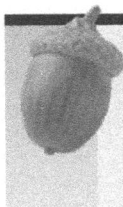

Dizziness
IN A NUTSHELL

Check medications.

Prescribe treatment.

Do teaching with patient and family.

CHAPTER 51

Hiccups

- **Irritation of the phrenic nerve on the neck or mediastinum**: most common
- **Irritation of the diaphragm from above**:
  - Lung carcinoma
  - Mesothelioma of the pleura
  - Carcinoma of the lower third of the esophagus
- **Irritation of the phrenic nerve from below**:
  - Carcinoma of the stomach
  - Abdominal carcinomatosis
  - Hepatomegaly
  - Uremia
- **Central, from within the brain itself**: occasional

Although relatively rare, this is a potentially distressing symptom. The length of time a patient must endure the hiccups, rather than the intensity of diaphragmatic contractions, causes the patient to be distressed.

Effect: Some patients liken the experience to "water torture."

INTERVENTIONS

Mild to Moderately Distressing Hiccups

- **Metoclopramide** (Reglan), 10 to 20 mg every 6 hours:
  - *May increase pain and/or nausea* in patients with GI obstructions
  - *Lowers seizure threshold*
- Peppermint water
- Mylanta

If Metoclopramide Is Ineffective After One or Two Doses

- **Chlorpromazine** (Thorazine), 25 to 50 g three or four times daily PO as needed:
  - Especially effective in hiccups that occur in conjunction with uremia

> *Warn patients about strong sedating effects and potential significant orthostatic hypotension effects.*

- If chlorpromazine is ineffective, you may suspect a central cause:
  - **Baclofen**, 5 mg PO three times daily; maximum, 80 mg per day
  - **Neurontin** (if unresponsive to Baclofen), 300 mg three times per day; may increase up to 1,800 mg per day

Teaching for Patients

- Advise the patient to anticipate drowsiness with sedating medications:
  - Do not drive or operate heavy machinery.
  - Use fall prevention measures.
  - Avoid postural hypotension: Move slowly when changing positions.

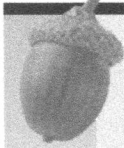

Hiccups
IN A NUTSHELL

Relatively rare but distressing symptom.

Increasing distress to patients with length of time.

Originates with phrenic nerve, diaphragm, or brain.

Monitor results and change treatments until effective relief of symptoms.

Teach patient and family about side effects.

CHAPTER 52

Fatigue

Fatigue is an overwhelming sense of tiredness or exhaustion.

Origin

- Normal early symptom of the dying process
- May be prominent complaint in cognitively intact:
    - Can rate it (0–10 scale or mild, moderate, severe)
- May be associated with depression

Fatigue may lead to **decreased ADLs and more or less sleep.**

Interventions

- Clarify impact on functional status and mood.
- Explore the meaning of the symptom to patient, family.
- Consider OT/PT with goal of improving quality of life vs. function.
- Consider gait training, positioning, and assistive devices for energy conservation.
- Consider treating contributory factors:
    - Anemia; electrolyte imbalance
    - Antidepressants, including methylphenidate

Teaching for Patients

- Give the patient permission to rest.
- Anticipate increased fatigue as time passes.
- Explain that fatigue is a normal part of the dying process.

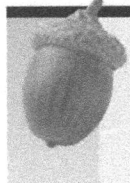

Fatigue
IN A NUTSHELL

Fatigue will lead to decreased ADLs.

Consider OT/PT.

Treat contributing factors.

CHAPTER 53

Anorexia

Origin

- **Normal symptom of the dying process**:
    - Results from diversion of oxygen-rich blood supply from digestive tract (nonessential for life under stress) to heart and brain

Effect

- **Relieves unnecessary burden of digestion** on stressed body systems
- **Triggers benefits of dehydration**:
    - Decreased workload for circulatory system
    - Decreased risk of edema or unwanted excessive secretions
    - Release of body's own Demerol-like endorphins

Interventions

- Rule out nonterminal causes:
    - Pain
    - Depression
    - Medications
    - Oral problems
    - Other GI problems
- Do workup, and prescribe treatments based on:
    - Benefits and burdens
    - Patient's prognosis
    - Preference
    - Goals

- Educate family.
- Address cultural, religious concerns.
- Encourage other ways to show love besides feeding.

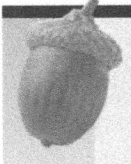

Anorexia
IN A NUTSHELL

Normal part of dying process

Weigh benefit vs. burden in treatment

Educate family

CHAPTER 54

Constipation

Origin

- **Common nonsubsiding effect of opioid use**

  > "The hand that writes the opioid order should write the bowel regimen."—Dame Cicely Saunders

- **Poor motility**
  - Dying process
  - Diabetes
  - Decreased activity
- **Dehydration**
- **Any medication with anticholinergic properties**:
  - Antidepressants
  - Cardiovascular medications
  - Antipsychotics

Effects

- **Agitation**
- **Delirium**
- **Vomiting**
- **Pain**
- **Anorexia**
- **Urinary retention**
- **New-onset incontinence**
- **Abdominal distension**
- May lead to **impaction**, evidenced by oozing diarrhea

Prevention

- Scheduled toileting, sitting up if possible
- Maintain evacuation every 2 to 3 days:
  - Clear GI secretions, desquamation, bacteria
- Prescribe laxative along with opioid pain medications
  - Senna-S, 1 to 4 PO twice daily (combination of senna and docusate)

Treatment

- Check rectum (+/– radiograph) for impaction.
- **Fiber** (psyllium) may help:
  - Will harm in setting of dehydration or poor motility
- **Fluid**: Increase water intake or keep fluid in gut with osmotic:
  - MiraLax (GlycoLax), lactulose, sorbitol
  - For some patients, sorbitol too sweet
- **Motility** (Mg salts, senna, bisacodyl, cascara):
  - Use senna *after* impaction/obstipation is cleared
  - Worse with opioids, anticholinergics, tricyclics, scopolamine, oxybutynin, promethazine, diphenhydramine, lithium, verapamil, bismuth, iron, aluminum, calcium
- **Lubrication** (DSS tabs, glycerin suppositories)

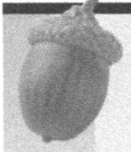

Constipation
IN A NUTSHELL

Common cause of many problems:

Anticipate when prescribing opioids.

Prevent when possible (i.e., bowel regimen).

Treat appropriately and aggressively.

CHAPTER 55

Delirium

FEATURES

Delirium is a **cognitive disorder**.

- Perception:
    - Visual and auditory illusions
    - Confusion
    - Hallucinations
    - Paranoia
- Thinking:
    - Disorganized
    - Incoherent
- Memory:
    - Disoriented to time

It is also an attention disorder of awareness and consciousness. It fluctuates during the day and is worse at night.

- **Sleep/wake cycle abnormalities:**
    - Sleep during the day
    - Agitated at night
- **Psychomotor abnormalities:**
    - Movements and speech: hypo- or hyperactive
    - Marked startle response
    - Emotions: apathy, depression, fear, rage

Delirium differentiates from dementia, in which:

- One is alert and aware of surroundings.
- There is defective knowledge of commonly known facts.
- There is no fluctuation as in delirium.
- Pharmacologic interventions usually are not indicated.

Origin

- **Cancer metastases to CNS and metabolic encephalopathy**:
    - Vital organ failure
    - Electrolyte abnormalities
    - Nutritional
- **Infection and sepsis**
- **Poor vascular perfusion**
- **Drug effects**:
    - Sedatives
    - Opiates
    - Antinauseants
    - Anticholinergics
    - Cimetidine
    - Reglan
    - Digoxin
    - Beta-blockers
    - Antiarrhythmics
    - Benzodiazepine
- **Paraneoplastic syndromes**

Management

- Consider change in narcotic agent.
- Reduce anxiety and disorientation by quiet, well-lit surroundings with familiar objects.
- Haldol:
    - 0.5 mg to 5 mg PO, two to three times daily, decreases agitation without sedation
    - Dose every 30 to 60 minutes as needed for rapid tranquilization of severely agitated patient
- Sometimes combining benzodiazepines (such as Ativan, 1 to 2 mg to start) with Haldol may be necessary for adequate relief.
- Seroquel may be used for those with extrapyramidal symptoms; start 25 mg twice daily; dosing range, 25 to 100 mg, two to three times daily.

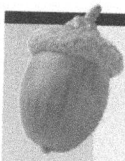

Delirium
IN A NUTSHELL

Cognitive and attention disorder

Sleep/wake cycle and psychomotor abnormalities

Differentiates from dementia:

Unaware of surroundings

Defective knowledge of common facts

Fluctuation of awareness/consciousness

CHAPTER 56

Diarrhea

EVALUATIONS

- **Medication related**:
  - Discontinue magnesium-based antacids (change to aluminum based)
  - Discontinue metoclopramide (Reglan)
- **Infection (particularly in AIDS)**:
  - Definitive treatment based on stool culture results
  - Ciprofloxacin (Cipro) + Metronidazole (Flagyl)
  - Octreotide (Somatostatin), 50 to 150 μg SC two to three times daily (carcinoid tumor)
- **Pseudomembranous colitis—consider recent antibiotics**:
  - Discontinue antibiotics (penicillins, sulfas, cephalosporins)
  - Metronidazole (Flagyl), 500 mg every 6 hours for 10 days
  - Probiotic: Culturelle, Florastor, yogurt, and so on.
- **Pancreatic insufficiency (steatorrhea)—check for pancreatic cancer**:
  - Pancrease MT, 1 to 3 capsules before meals; dosing varies
  - Pancreatin, 1 to 2 tablets before meals; dosing varies
- **Colitis—check for bloody stools**:
  - Steroid enema
  - Sulfasalazine (Azulfidine), 1 g three to four times daily
- **Idiopathic**:
  - Metamucil
  - Kaopectate
  - Questran, 1 packet twice daily
  - Diphenoxylate/Atropine (Lomotil), 2 capsules two to four times daily

- Loperamide (Imodium):
    - For control of **diarrhea and abdominal cramping**: 2 to 4 mg PO every 6 hours

TEACHING

Diet

- Liquids in, liquids out: No treatment; maintain hydration:
    - Water (if given alone will induce electrolyte disturbances after 2 to 5 days)
    - Clear soups and juices
    - Gatorade
    - 7UP
    - Kool-Aid
    - Ginger ale
- Lactose intolerance: Eliminate dairy products

Skin Problems

- **Protective barrier important**:
    - A & D ointment
    - Desitin ointment
    - Uniderm ointment
    - Vaseline

Reintroducing Solids in Prudent Stepwise Fashion

1. Begin with full liquids.
2. If well tolerated over 12 to 36 hours, progress to soft diet.
3. Carefully progress to regular diet.
4. If well tolerated over the next 24 hours, resume daily bowel regimen by half to third of regular dose, then increase gradually.
5. If diarrhea reappears, repeat steps 1 through 4.

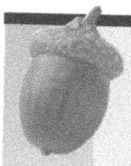

Diarrhea
IN A NUTSHELL

Evaluate cause.

Stop medications that may be causing it, including bowel regimen.

Prescribe appropriate treatment.

Do teaching with patient and family related to diet, skin care, and reintroduction of bowel regimen.

CHAPTER 57

Incontinence

Causes

- **Normal part of dying process**
- **Other causes include**:
    - Local tumor effects
    - Drug and radiation side effects
    - Infection
- **Treat if symptomatic only** (dysuria, etc.):
    - Metabolic consequences with polyuria
    - Diabetes mellitus, hypercalcemia, and so on
    - Debility, bladder spasm, detrusor instability
    - Anatomic or neurologic damage
    - Retention with overflow
    - Anxiety

Treatment

- **Antibiotic, if indicated**
- **Change diuretic regimen**
- **Drug measures to decrease detrusor irritability**:
    - Urispas (flavoxate), 100 to 200 mg three to four times daily
    - Ditropan (oxybutynin), 5 mg every 6 hours as needed
    - Tofranil (imipramine) or Elavil, 10 to 50 mg at bedtime or twice daily
    - Vesicare, 5 to 10 mg daily
    - Sanctura, 20 mg twice daily
- **Insert indwelling catheter**

Teaching with Caregivers

- **Increased risk for skin problems—protective barrier important**:
  - A & D ointment
  - Desitin ointment
  - Uniderm ointment
  - Vaseline
- **Catheter care:**
  - Keep clean—cleanse away from patient.
  - Keep bag attached to catheter at all times.
  - Keep bag below the level of the bladder.
  - *Do not attach bag to bed or wheelchair if patient is ambulatory!*
  - Observe patient, not urine, for signs of possible urinary tract infection.

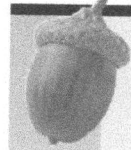

Incontinence
IN A NUTSHELL

Evaluate cause.

Treat, if appropriate.

Insert indwelling catheter:

Protects skin.

Decreases patient's anxiety related to toileting.

Relieves caregiver burden.

Decreases patient's discomfort related to changing incontinence products.

Do teaching with caregivers related to skin care and catheter care.

CHAPTER 58

Depression

The usual symptoms and signs of depression:

- **May be confused with or masked by symptoms and signs of disease.**
- **May be masked by cognitive impairment:**
  - Keep high index of suspicion.
  - Beware: "Of course, she's depressed."
  - Explore the meaning of patient's feelings, especially worthlessness, hopelessness.
  - Distinguish preparatory grief from depression.

Management

- **Attend to whatever is distressing patient:**
  - Pain, other symptoms, social issues
- **Attend to cultural factors.**
- **Provide social, emotional, spiritual support.**
- **Enhance control.**
- **Encourage activities.**
- **Consider psychology referral.**
- **Consider antidepressants.**

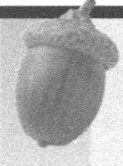

Depression
IN A NUTSHELL

Evaluate cause.

Attend to whatever is distressing patient.

Consider antidepressants.

CHAPTER 59

Nonhealing Wounds

NONHEALING CHRONIC WOUNDS

When the underlying etiology does not respond to treatment and/or the demands of treatment are beyond the patient's endurance or stamina, there is a need for communication.

> "This inability to achieve complete wound closure or, in some cases, prevent the occurrence of skin breakdown is contrary to most patients' and families' expectations."

Assessment of Chronic Wounds

- **Healing likelihood—no perfect formula**:
  - Etiology: pressure, venous, arterial, diabetic/neuropathic
  - Previous treatments
  - Compliance
  - Overall health status
  - Co-morbidities
  - Nutritional status
  - Osteomyelitis

Palliative Care Goals for Chronic Wounds

- **Complement curative goals**: *not* either/or
- **Focus on quality-of-life issues**:
  - Stabilize the wound.
  - Reduce pain (e.g., from dressing changes).
  - Reduce bacterial burden.
  - Reduce exudates.
  - Eliminate odor.

Principles of Care

- **Relieve pressure:**
    - Frequent repositioning and/or low-air-loss mattress
    - Elevate extremities *off* mattress, if possible
- **Do not massage a pressure area.**
- **Remember, open wounds must be kept moist to heal**.
- **Provide nutritional support, if prognosis warrants:**
    - Protein supplement
    - Multivitamins
    - Iron
    - Vitamin C, 500 mg three times daily
    - Zinc, 220 mg two times daily
- **Consider Foley catheter.**

Odor Control

- **Odor elimination:**
    - Débridement (mechanical or enzymatic)
    - Antibiotics (topical or oral), especially metronidazole gel for anaerobes
    - Papain-urea-chlorophyllin copper sodium: Panafil
- **Odor minimizers:**
    - Charcoal and/or baking soda–based topicals
    - Kitty litter placed under the bed

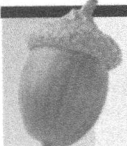

Wounds
IN A NUTSHELL

Relieve pressure.

Assess likelihood of healing and goals, especially palliation, when prescribing treatment.

Eliminate odor.

Consider Foley catheter.

CHAPTER 60

Pruritus

The symptom of itching: An uncomfortable sensation leading to the urge to scratch. Scratching may result in secondary infection.

Causes of Pruritus

- Allergy
- Infection
- Jaundice
- Chronic renal disease
- Lymphoma
- Skin irritation

Topical Treatment

- 0.1% Triamcinolone cream
- 1.0% Hydrocortisone cream
- Fluorinated steroid creams (Synalar, Lidex)
- Xylocaine jelly 2%

Systemic Treatment

- Antihistamine:
    - Hydroxyzine (Atarax), 25 to 50 mg four times per day
    - Diphenhydramine (Benadryl), 25 to 50 mg four times per day
    - Cyproheptadine (Periactin), 4 mg four times per day
- Dexamethasone, 4 mg PO daily to twice daily, or methylprednisolone taper (Medrol Dosepak)

- Candidiasis:
    - Miconazole (Micatin) 2%, topically
    - Ketoconazole (Nizoral), 200 mg daily
    - Fluconazole (Diflucan), 200 to 400 mg daily
- Jaundice:
    - Cholestyramine (Questran), 1 packet two to three times daily
- Herpes zoster:
    - Domeboro soaks
    - Acyclovir (Zovirax) 5% ointment
    - Acyclovir (Zovirax), 200 mg five times daily
- Mites:
    - Kildane (Kwell) lotion and shampoo
    - Crotamiton (Eurax) lotion and shampoo

Teaching for the Family and Caregivers

- **Relieve dry skin**
- Cool humidified air
- Avoid hot baths
- Avoid irritants and soap
- Topical treatment
- Lubrication:
    - Eucerin cream
    - Alpha-Keri lotion
    - Nutraderm bath oil
    - Anti-itch lotion: Gold Bond, Aveeno
    - Cornstarch and baking soda tepid water bath
- **Prevent clothing irritation**:
    - Cotton clothing and bed linens
    - Rinse with white vinegar to remove excessive soap

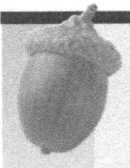

Pruritus
IN A NUTSHELL

Nontreatment can lead to secondary infection.

Treatment should be directed at the cause; may be a combination of systemic and topical.

CHAPTER 61

Insomnia

Sleeplessness: Chronic inability to sleep or to remain asleep throughout the night.

Causes of Insomnia

- Unrelieved pain
- Leg cramps
- Night sweats
- Idiopathic

Treatment

- Unrelieved pain: See chapter on pain control
- Leg cramps:
  - Quinine, 325 mg at bedtime
  - Neurontin, 300 mg once or twice daily. Titrate up to 1,200 mg per day if needed
- Night sweats:
  - Indomethacin (Indocin), 50 mg at bedtime
- Idiopathic:
  - Diphenhydramine (Benadryl), 50 to 100 mg at bedtime
  - Ambien, 5 to 10 mg at bedtime as needed
  - Lorazepam (Ativan), 0.5 to 1 mg at bedtime up to 4 mg
  - Alprazolam (Xanax), 0.25 to 0.5 mg at bedtime up to 2 mg
  - Trazodone, 25 to 50 mg at bedtime
  - Temazepam, 15 to 30 mg at bedtime

Teaching for the Family and Caregivers

- **Fear**:
    - Explore feelings through active listening.
    - Don't leave the patient alone.
    - Review life; reminisce.
- **Environment**:
    - Make consistent for the patient.
    - Decrease stimulation; keep room quiet; limit visitors.
    - Try relaxation techniques:
        - Light massage
        - Back rubs
        - Night light
        - Hot drink (milk, cocoa, alcohol)
- **Sleep patterns**:
    - Encourage consistent routines.
    - Understand changes that are typical for the dying patient.

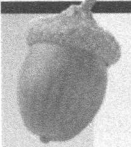

Insomnia
IN A NUTSHELL

Treat the cause, if known.

Explore the feelings of the patient.

Use pharmaceutical and nonpharmaceutical interventions.

Educate the family.

SECTION 7 BIBLIOGRAPHY

1. Storey P, Knight C. *Hospice/Palliative Care Training for Physicians, A Self-Study Program.* Glenview, Ill: American Academy of Hospice and Palliative Medicine; 2003.
2. Storey P, Knight C, Schonwetter R. *Pocket Guide to Hospice/Palliative Medicine.* Glenview, Ill: American Academy of Hospice and Palliative Medicine; 2003.
3. Swagerty D, Johnson M. *Primer for Hospice & Palliative Care Medicine,* Rockford, Ill: Hospice Care of America; 2005.

CHAPTER 62

Nightmares

Patients often have poor sleep quality as they approach the end of life, and nightmares (vivid and **terrifying dreams** in which one is **abruptly awakened** from sleep) are common. Nightmares occur almost exclusively during **REM** (rapid eye movement) sleep (1).

CAUSES

- **Medications**: sedative/hypnotics, antidepressants, benzodiazepines, beta-blockers, and others
- **Anxiety** or other **psychiatric** conditions: delirium, mood disorder, posttraumatic stress disorder, and so on
- **CNS disorders**: brain metastasis or infections
- **Systemic disorders**: infection, hypoglycemia, high ammonia levels (liver failure), and so on

TREATMENTS

Once the **cause** is determined, treatment can be effective. However, in palliative patients, it is often not practical to treat the underlying cause (brain metastases, etc.), and the symptoms must be treated.

- **Nonpharmacological** treatments: psychotherapy, behavior techniques, desensitization, and so on.
- Clonazepam (Klonopin), 0.5 to 1.0 mg at bedtime (2)
- Risperidone (Risperdal), 0.5 to 2 mg PO at bedtime (3)
- Olanzapine (Zyprexa), 5 mg PO; increase to a maximum of 20 mg at bedtime (4)
- Cyproheptadine (Periactin), 4 to 8 mg PO three times per day or at bedtime
- Topiramate (Topamax), 25 mg two times per day; titrate 25 mg per week to maximum of 200 mg two times per day.

- Benzodiazepines and tricyclic antidepressants may suppress REM sleep and prevent nightmares. However, they may have a paradoxical effect and should be used with caution.

- **Note**: Trazodone **does not** suppress REM activity.

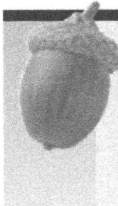

Nightmares
IN A NUTSHELL

Only nightmares that are disturbing to the patient need to be treated.

Most treatment of nightmares near the end of life is palliative, with a goal to ensure restful sleep.

REFERENCES

1. Pagel JF. Nightmares and disorders of dreaming, Am Fam Physician. 2000;61:2037–2042, 2044.
2. Schenck CH, Mahowald MW. REM sleep parasomnias. Neurol Clin. 1996;14:697–720.
3. Stanovic JK, James KA, Vandevere CA. The effectiveness of risperidone on acute stress symptoms in adult burn patient: a preliminary retrospective pilot study. J Burn Care Rehabil. 2001;22:210–213.
4. Labbate LA, Douglas S. Olanzapine for nightmares and sleep disturbance in posttraumatic stress disorder (PTSD). Can J Psychiatry. 2000;45:667–668.

Pain Control

CHAPTER 63

Myths About Opioid Use

Chronic pain, especially in the elderly and in end-of-life care, is notoriously **undertreated** (1). Physicians, nurses, and patients all have misconceptions about the use of the most effective available class of medications for treating pain—the opioids. This chapter provides the correct responses to the most common myths about morphine and other opioids.

Myth: Opioids Cause Severe Respiratory Depression

- Clinically significant respiratory depression is **extremely rare** when patients receive appropriate doses of opioids, even in patients with respiratory diseases, including COPD, CHF, and lung cancer (2).

- Patients **do not go from awake and talking to dead** without going through various stages of sedation first. Patients become significantly comatose before respiratory depression is noted.

- If a patient on a consistent dose of opioid shows deterioration, such as weakness, confusion, cool extremities, and slowed respirations, suspect increased disease.

Myth: Using Opioids Leads to Addiction

- Addiction is an **extremely rare** occurrence when opioids are used in patients with pain (3).

> **Think of it this way: Pain acts as an antidote to morphine. When pain is present, it soaks up the opioid and the patient gets very few effects such as addiction, tolerance, or withdrawal.**

- When pain is reduced by radiation or other treatments, opioids can be **tapered rapidly** without withdrawal symptoms in the vast majority of patients. This fact can be used to assure patients that they are not addicted.

- **Tolerance is** an **unusual** problem. Once a patient's pain is controlled at a certain dose of medication, it may stay the same dose for years. If a patient is well

controlled at a consistent dose, and pain escalates, suspect increasing disease
rather than tolerance (see Table 7)!

TABLE 7

Important Definitions

Tolerance: Increasing dose of medication to get the same effect (alcohol, laxatives)
Physical dependence: Withdrawal symptoms when suddenly stopping medication (beta-blockers, corticosteroids, benzodiazepines, clonidine)
Addiction: Continued use of anything, in spite of harm. Overwhelming involvement in the acquisition and use of drugs for nonmedical purposes (diversion). Note: The presence of tolerance or physical dependence does not prove addiction!

Myth: Taking Opioids Means You Are a Weak or Bad Person

• Opioids are just another medication used for pain. Because they are sometimes abused, their legitimate use for pain has become stigmatized. (Doesn't this category also include guns, fire, even airplanes in the hands of terrorists?)

Myth: Opioids Cause Imminent Death in the Severely Ill

• The terminal patient may relax and die after a dose of opioid for pain, but it is the disease that has killed the patient, not the dose of medication.

• "I don't want to be the last person to give the morphine." Well, someone is going to give the last everything—the last gelatin, the last drink of water, and the last haircut! It is an honor to be involved in keeping a dying patient comfortable!

Myth: Opioids Damage the Body

• Opioids are very **safe**. The American Geriatric Society has determined that opioids are safer for the elderly than ibuprofen!

• There are no dosage warnings in liver, renal, or pulmonary disease.

Myth: Opioids have Severe Side Effects

• **Nausea** is the most common side effect and occurs in about 30% of patients when they initially take opioids (2). However, nausea usually **resolves** over **3 to 5 days** of continued treatment. This does not indicate an allergy to the opioids!

• Other transient side effects include sedation, confusion, dizziness, dysphonia, itching, urinary retention, and others. Again, these all tend to resolve over several days if the medication is continued.

• Constipation is the only side effect that will not go away!

CONCLUSION

Opioids are very **safe, effective, and well-tolerated medications for pain**. The myths cited in this chapter should not be barriers to patients receiving good pain control at the end of life (4)!

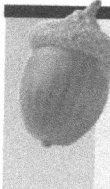

Myths of Opioid Use
IN A NUTSHELL

Clinically **significant respiratory depression is rare** at appropriate doses.

Addiction is a rare outcome in treating pain at end of life.

Opioids have a stigma but are excellent medications for pain.

Morphine given to the terminally ill with the intent of pain control is not dangerous and **should not be withheld** because of fear of imminent death.

Opioids are very **safe** when given appropriately.

Side effects, except constipation, are usually **transient** and do not mean the patient is allergic to opioids.

REFERENCES

1. Foley KM. Acute and chronic cancer pain syndromes. In: Doyle D, Hanks G, Cherny NI, et al., eds. *Oxford Textbook of Palliative Medicine*. 3rd ed. New York: Oxford University Press; 2004:299.
2. Storey P, Knight CF. Alleviating Psychological and Spiritual Pain in the Terminally Ill. UNIPAC Two, *Hospice/Palliative Care Training for Physicians*. 2nd ed. Glenview, Illinois: American Academy of Hospice and Palliative Medicine; 2003:25.
3. Whitecar PS, Jonas AP, Clasen ME. Managing pain in the dying patient. Am Fam Physician. 2000;61:755–764.
4. Joranson DE, Ryan KM, Gilson AM, et al. Trends in medical use and abuse of opioid analgesics. JAMA. 2000;283:1710–1714.

CHAPTER 64

Legal Liability of Undertreating Pain

The **fear of legal sanctions** has traditionally been one of the major factors why physicians and other clinicians undertreat pain (1). The majority of physicians still fear regulatory scrutiny from federal, state, and local agencies when using high doses of opioids to control intractable pain. However, the **undertreatment of pain** is now becoming recognized as a **major public health problem**. As a result, health care providers are beginning to see public expectations change, and they now **face possible legal action for not treating pain adequately** (2).

EVIDENCE OF CHANGE

Public policy and **legal precedent** regarding the use of controlled substances for treatment of pain is **changing**. New policies are being shaped by **clinical guidelines**, a preponderance of **sound scientific evidence**, and **case law**. Although the legal aspects of pain treatment are still in the development phase, there are many indications that **undertreatment of pain will soon be considered a greater legal issue** than the fear of overtreatment:

- 1998: The first case where a **physician** was sued and **found guilty** of "reckless negligence" and elder abuse for undertreating pain occurred in the state of California (*Bergman v Chin*).

- 2003: The Medical Board of California initiated action against a physician for **undertreating pain** in a skilled nursing facility (*Tomlinson v Whitney*).

- Since 1990 there has been a **dramatic increase in state legislation** governing the treatment of intractable pain (3).

- 2004: An analysis tracking the use of opioids from 1997 to 2002 showed a **dramatic increase**—400% for oxycodone—in the **medical use of opioids for pain control** (4).

- **Cooperation between** the **Drug Enforcement Administration (DEA)**, **medical organizations**, and **national experts** in pain and addiction is continuing.

- Overwhelming **scientific evidence** and research supports the aggressive treatment of pain, and is dispelling many of the previous myths about addiction and the dangers of opioids.

- Several justices of the **U.S. Supreme Court** have written opinions that support the use of pain medication even in doses that could possibly hasten death, as long as the physician's **intent** is to relieve pain and suffering and not to end the patient's life (5).

- The increasing **political influence** of the savvy aging baby boomers is supporting good pain control (6).

THE PITFALLS

Because **legal precedent is slow to change**, today's clinicians still face a number of challenges when attempting to treat pain properly:

- As the medical use of opioids for pain control has increased, so has the **abuse and diversion** of those drugs.

- Because of the increase in diversion, government and law enforcement agencies are focusing again on the **prescribing habits of physicians**.

- An **occasional** high-profile case has been filed where **criminal charges** have been brought against a physician for overtreatment of pain, resulting in an alleged hastened death.

- There is a **perception** that those with the moral charge of adequately treating pain are **at odds** with the agencies that are protecting society from illicit drug use.

WHAT TO DO

Clinicians can be sued for overtreating pain or undertreating pain! But this is America: **Anyone can be sued for anything!** Until public policy and regulatory agencies work out the answer, **good pain control for our patients is still a moral responsibility**. Here are a few tips on how to avoid legal action:

- **Improve** your own **skills and knowledge** in pain assessment and treatment through Continuing Medical Education (CME) or other opportunities.

- **Assess** each patient well for pain management and have a documented treatment plan. Have a **good history and physical (H&P) and records** of the patient's psychosocial and physical function.

- **Reassess** the patient frequently and evaluate the progress toward the treatment goals, with emphasis on function.

- **Document** the discussion of **risks and benefits** (informed consent) that has occurred with the patient or the family.

- **Refer** to a pain specialist or ask for **consultation** on difficult cases, such as patients with a previous history of substance abuse.

- Keep a **good record** of all pain medications, including the date, dosage, number of pills, and refills if applicable.

- **Be alert** to drug-seeking behaviors, but also be aware of pseudo-addiction (see Chapter 81).
- Be **knowledgeable** and **compliant** with all **controlled substance laws**.
- Do what is **best for the patient**!

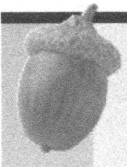

Legal Liability of Undertreating Pain
IN A NUTSHELL

Public policy seems to be changing in favor of **treating pain** adequately.

Scientific evidence and the **medical literature** favor **treating pain** aggressively.

Because legal precedent is slow to change, there are **still a few pitfalls** in pain treatment.

Fear of legal sanctions is **not a good reason** for failing to treat pain appropriately.

Be **knowledgeable** and **document** well.

Not treating pain well comes close to **inflicting it!**

REFERENCES

1. Hoffman DE, Tarzian AJ. Achieving the right balance in oversight of physician opioid prescribing for pain: the role of state medical boards. J Law Med Ethics. 2003;31:21–40.
2. Fishman SM. Legal aspects in pain medicine for primary care physicians. Supplement to Family Practice News. New York: Academy for Healthcare Education Inc.; 2006. Available at: www.AHECME.com.
3. Pain & Policy Studies Group. Madison: University of Wisconsin/WHO Collaborating Center; 2006. Available at: www.painpolicy.wisc.edu. Updated January 2007.
4. Gilson AM, Ryan KM, Joranson DE, et al. A reassessment of trends in medical use and abuse of opioid analgesics and implications for diversion control: 1997–2002. J Pain Symptom Manage. 2004;28:176–188.
5. Meisel JD, Synder L, Quill T. Seven legal barriers to end-of-life care: Myths, realities and grains of truth. JAMA. 2000;284:2495–2501.
6. Warm EJ, Weissman DE. The legal liability of under-treatment of pain. *Fast Facts and Concepts # 63*. Milwaukee: Medical College of Wisconsin. Available at: http://www.eperc.mcw.edu/fastFact/ff_63.htm. Assessed April 9, 2006.

CHAPTER 65

Principles of Pain Management

Most **pain** experienced at the end of life can be **managed** in a relatively **simple and straightforward** manner (1). Do not be afraid to treat pain **aggressively and persistently**. This chapter describes the general principles that apply to pain management.

STAY AHEAD OF THE PAIN

Pain is like fire: It is much easier to extinguish when it is small. Chronic pain should be treated **around the clock** rather than allowing for periods of subtherapeutic treatment with exacerbations of the pain and then trying to catch up. Here are some methods for staying ahead of pain (2):

- Prescribe short-acting pain medications in **doses that make pharmacological sense**. For example, the maximum analgesic effect of short-acting medications such as codeine, hydrocodone, and oxycodone is 4 hours. So don't give them every 6 or 12 hours.

- Chronic pain almost always requires **scheduled dosing**, which maintains a steady state of medication and provides constant relief while minimizing side effects.

- **Beware of as needed (PRN)** orders because pain medications are generally not given in the hospital or nursing home until the pain peaks.

- Use **long-acting preparations** to maintain serum levels: for example, Morphine SR, MS Contin, Oxycodone SR, or OxyContin, given orally every 8 to 12 hours. The Fentanyl patch lasts 48 to 72 hours. For parenteral administration, use continuous administration (patient-controlled analgesia [PCA] pump).

- Use **dose escalation** if the pain is not controlled.

- Involve the patient in their pain control: **education**.

PROVIDE A BREAKTHROUGH DOSE

Along with the long-acting baseline pain medication, always provide the patient with a short-acting dose to use for breakthrough pain (3). This should be **10% to 20% of the total daily dose** given PRN for pain.

- This short-acting dose may be used before certain **activities**, like dressing changes, bathing, and so on, and prevents pain from escalating.
- If a patient is using frequent doses of breakthrough medications, then the baseline or long-acting medication needs to be reevaluated and possibly increased.

ESCALATE THE DOSE

If the pain is not controlled, escalate the dose (see Dose Escalation):

- For **mild pain**, increase the dose by **25%**.
- For **moderate pain**, increase the dose by **25% to 50%**.
- For **severe pain**, increase the dose by **50% to 100%**.
- **Be knowledgeable** about the onset, peak, and duration of the specific pain medication ordered.
- **Monitor** and reassess the patient frequently.

MEDICATION CHOICES

The World Health Organization (WHO) recommends a very simple but effective **three-step approach** for treating pain (4). The medications used depend on the severity of the pain: mild, moderate, and severe. Most clinicians start at step 2 or 3 if patients present in moderate to severe pain (5).

- Step 1. Acetaminophen (maximum daily adult dose: 4 g), NSAIDs, or COX-2.
- Step 2. When pain is not controlled at step 1, add a weak opioid, such as codeine, hydrocodone, or oxycodone.

TABLE 8

Adjuvants to Opioid Therapy (2)

Adjuvant	Common Indications
Alpha-blocker (clonidine)	Neuropathic pain
Anticonvulsants (gabapentin, tiagabine)	Neuropathic or postherpetic neuralgia
Antihistamines (diphenhydramine)	Nausea, pruritus, or anxiety
Benzodiazepines (clonazepam, diazepam, lorazepam)	Anxiety or myoclonus
Corticosteroids (dexamethasone, prednisone)	Bone pain, nerve compression, or increased intracranial pressure
NSAIDs and COX-2 inhibitors (celecoxib, ibuprofen, naproxen)	Musculoskeletal pain
Tricyclic antidepressants (amitriptyline, desipramine, nortriptyline)	Neuropathic pain or postherpetic neuralgia

Adopted from WHO, 1990.

- Step 3. If pain persists, got to the next level by starting morphine, hydromorphone, or fentanyl.

- Adjuvant can be added at any stage to enhance analgesia or to treat certain conditions that exacerbate pain, such as bone metastasis. Adjuvants include corticosteroids, antihistamines, benzodiazepines, NSAIDs, tricyclic antidepressants, certain anticonvulsants, and others (see Table 8).

- Avoid meperidine (Demerol) and the mixed-agonist antagonists. See Figure 9.

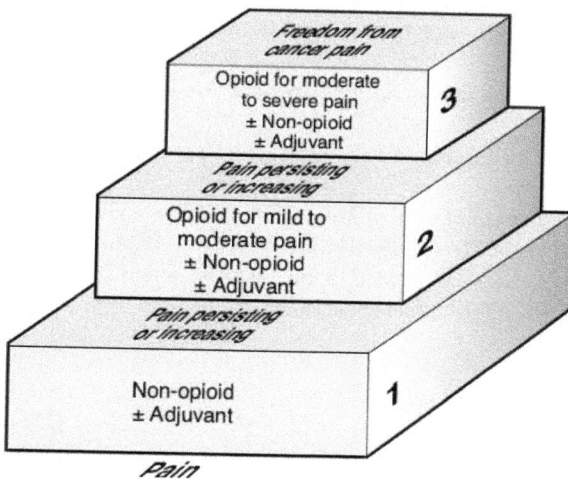

FIGURE 9 ●

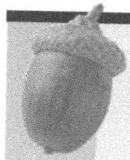

Principles of Pain Management
IN A NUTSHELL

Treat pain aggressively and persistently.

Stay ahead of the pain: Use scheduled dosing for chronic pain.

Use **long-acting medications** to maintain a steady serum level, and provide **breakthrough doses** (10–20% of daily dose) for pain exacerbations.

Escalate the dose if needed (mild, 25%; moderate, 25% to 50%; severe, 50% to 100%)

Chose medications based on the type and severity of the pain: **WHO ladder.**

Use a multidrug approach by combining opioids with nonopioid **adjuvants.**

Use the **oral route** unless contraindicated.

ADMINISTERING PAIN MEDICATIONS

- Use the least invasive route for pain medications. We often forget that the **oral route** almost always works. Concentrated morphine drops (Roxanol) can be given orally in most conscious patients. The oral route is also the most cost efficient.

- Manage the **side effects** of opioids aggressively.

REFERENCES

1. Storey P, Knight CF. Alleviating psychological and spiritual pain in the terminally ill, UNI-PAC Two. *Hospice/Palliative Care Training for Physicians*. 2nd ed. Glenview, Illinois: American Academy of Hospice and Palliative Medicine 2003:15.
2. Pain Management Partnership. *Analgesic Reference Guide, 2005*. Kansas City: University of Kansas School of Medicine. 2005.
3. Whitecar PS, Jonas AP, Clasen ME. Managing pain in the dying patient. Am Fam Physician. 2000;61:755–764.
4. *WHO Ladder: Cancer Pain Relief and Palliative Care*. Technical Report Series 804. Geneva: World Health Organization; 1990.
5. Jacoz A, Carr DB, Payne R, et al. *Management of Cancer Pain*. Clinical Practice Guideline, 1994. Washington, DC: US. Department of Health and Human Services—Public Health Service. Health Services/Technology Assessment Text (HSTAT) can be found online at http:www.ncbi.nlm.nih.gov/books/bv.fcgi?rid=hstat6.chapter.18803.

CHAPTER 66

Assessment of Pain

Pain is the most feared element encountered by patients near the end of life. Most patients are less afraid of death than they are of dying with prolonged intractable pain (1). However, we must remember that pain and "suffering" are not the same. Emotional, social, and spiritual pain can cause a great deal of suffering and may be confused with physical pain.

Assessment for pain or potential pain, therefore, is a **priority** in palliative care. A good pain assessment includes the steps outlined here.

Gold standard: "Pain is what the patient tells you it is!"

GENERAL HISTORY OF THE PAIN

Pain is subjective; it should be considered to be whatever the patient says it is (2). Pain occurs in the context of a person's life, and his or her report of pain is modified by fears, hopes, spiritual beliefs, social factors, and economic realities. Here are some general characteristics to help identify the pain:

- **Location**: "Where is the pain?" "All over" is an acceptable answer, although this description might tip the scales in favor of emotional or spiritual pain rather than physical.
- **Duration**: "How long have you had the pain?"
- Temporal **pattern**: "Does it hurt all the time?" Or, "When does it bother you the most?"
- **Modifiers**: "What makes it better and worse?"

QUALITY OF PAIN

Physical pain can have the following origins (3):

- **Somatic** (muscle pain): Dull/aching type of pain that is well localized. Examples include a muscle strain, contusion, fractured bone, or bone metastasis.

- **Visceral** (from a hollow viscus or encapsulated organ): Deep, dull, cramping, sharp, colicky, type of pain that is vague and not well localized (may include referred pain).
- **Neuropathic** (nerve pain): Lancinating, stabbing, burning, numbing, or shooting electrical pain. This type of pain often follows a dermatome or nerve distribution pattern.
- **Mixed** or complex pain: This includes multiple causes for pain, such as neuropathic pain plus spiritual pain. Treatment will be disappointing unless these can be separated out.

INTENSITY OF PAIN

Although **pain assessment scales** are often consuming, they probably give the best results as to pain intensity. The numerical scale (0, no pain, and 10, the worst possible pain), FACES, or similar scales are all available. However, the use of a specific type of scale may be less important than ensuring that the scale used has these characteristics (4):

- **Completed by the patient** and not someone else.
- **Flexible** enough to be adapted to the specific needs of a particular patient.
- **Simple** enough to be used routinely and regularly.
- The same scale used on the same patient **consistently**.

TREATMENTS

Most everyone in pain has tried something for pain relief—drug or nondrug. Responses to treatment are also important. Questions to ask include the following:

- For drug therapy: Ask about quality of pain relief—for example the pain goes from a 9/10 to a 4/10. Ask how long it takes for the medication to take effect and how long the relief lasts.
- What other approaches have been tried? Blocks? Acupuncture? Herbs? Magnets?
- Has a pain workup been done at a pain clinic or by a pain specialist?

IMPACT OF PAIN ON ACTIVITIES OF DAILY LIVING

It is important to find out how pain is affecting the patient's function and activities of daily living (ADLs). Does the pain interfere with:

- **Sleep**? Lack of sleep may be interfering with the patient's general health.
- **Eating**? Is weight loss secondary to pain?
- **Mobility**? Sometimes treating pain and allowing just enough mobility for the patient to sit on the front porch in the sun will also cure the symptoms of depression.
- **Mood**/emotional response?

GOALS FOR PAIN RELIEF

What are the patient's **goals** for pain relief? Is it to be completely pain free? Or is the expectation to lower the pain intensity from 9/10 to 4/10? Most patients do not expect to be totally pain free but want to have a significant reduction in their pain. Are there **functional expectations**?

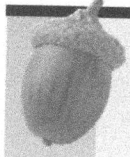

Assessment of Pain
IN A NUTSHELL

Pain is whatever the patient says it is!

Determine the **location, duration, temporal pattern, and modifiers** (worse/better).

Quality of pain: Somatic, visceral, neuropathic, or complex/mixed.

Intensity: Use pain intensity scale appropriate for the patient.

Treatments: What has been tried?

What impact has the pain had on **function**?

What are the **patient's goals** in pain relief?

Don't forget **spiritual, social,** and **emotional** pain.

REFERENCES

1. Bruera E, Kim HN. Cancer pain. JAMA. 2003;290:2476–2479.
2. Whitecar PS, Jonas AP, Clasen ME. Managing pain in the dying patient. Am Fam Physician. 2000;61:755–764.
3. Weissman DE. Pain assessment—teaching outline. In: *Improving End-of-Life Care, a Faculty Development Course Book for Medical Educators.* Milwaukee: The Medical College of Wisconsin; 2001.
4. Storey P, Knight CF. Alleviating psychological and spiritual pain in the terminally ill. UNIPAC Two, *Hospice/Palliative Care Training for Physicians.* 2nd ed. Glenview, Illinois: American Academy of Hospice and Palliative Medicine, 2003:18.

CHAPTER 67

Converting One Opioid to Another (Equianalgesic Dosing)

One of the very unique characteristics of opioids is that an **equal analgesic effect** can be achieved from **every opioid** if given in the proper dose. In other words, an equal pain relief can be obtained from hydrocodone (Lortab, Vicodin, Norco, etc.), morphine (MSIR, MS Contin, Roxanol, etc.), oxycodone (OxyIR, Percocet, OxyContin, etc.), hydromorphone (Dilaudid), and so on, if given in appropriate doses. This makes it very **easy to switch** from one opioid to another and from one route of administration to another.

Equianalgesic values are readily available in manuals and pain pocket guides (see Table 9 and appendix). The conversion calculations are very simple once they are mastered, but they have not been taught to most of today's practicing clinicians (1).

> **Example:** 30 mg of oral morphine is the same as 10 mg of IV morphine, which is also the same as 7.5 mg of oral hydromorphone, or 30 mg of oral hydrocodone.

CROSS TOLERANCE

When switching from one opioid to another opioid (not just the formulation, such as from MSIR to MS Contin), most experts recommend **reducing the new dose by 50%** because of the possibility of **cross tolerance** (2). The theory is that patients may have developed some tolerance to their old opioid, and therefore they may become overdosed on the new opioid even though the dose is equal. Tolerance seems to develop to side effects more than to the analgesic effect of opioids, so patients who are tolerant to the sedation, for example, on one opioid may become acutely sedated when the equal dose of another opioid is started.

However, **clinical judgment** is needed (3):

- If the patient's pain is poorly controlled, less dose reduction (i.e., 25%) is indicated.
- If the patient has a history of adverse effects, a greater dose reduction (i.e., 75%) may be indicated.

TABLE 9

Opioid Equianalgesic Doses (Approximate Guidelines Only)

Opioid	Oral Dose	Parenteral Dose
Morphine (MSIR, Roxanol, MS Contin, Kadian, Oramorph, Avinza, etc.)	30 mg	10 mg
Hydromorphone (Dilaudid)	7.5 mg	1.5 mg
Oxycodone (OxyIR, Roxicodone, Percocet, Roxicet, Percodan, OxyFast, etc.)	20–30 mg	N/A
Hydrocodone (Lortab, Lorcet, Norco, Vicodin)	30 mg	N/A
Fentanyl (Actiq oral lollipop, Duragesic patch)	Unknown	0.1 mg (100 µg) IV 0.015 mg (15 µg) transdermal patch
Meperidine (Demerol) (not recommended for chronic pain!)	300 mg	100 mg

SAMPLE CALCULATIONS

Morphine is the standard for pain control. Therefore, it is easiest to first convert all opioid doses into a dose of oral morphine. Then that dose can be converted into any other dose of any opioid (4).

Changing the Route of Administration

- A cancer patient is taking MS Contin 60 mg orally twice daily at home for pain. She is hospitalized for a procedure and made NPO. What dose of IV morphine will be needed to give her the same pain relief?
    - Figure out the 24-hour dose of oral morphine: 60 mg × 2/day = 120 mg/day.
    - Look up the equianalgesic value of morphine: 30 mg of oral is equal to 10 mg of IV (IV morphine is three times stronger!).
    Do the math:

$$\frac{30 \text{ mg oral morphine}}{120 \text{ mg oral morphine}} = \frac{10 \text{ mg of IV morphine}}{X \text{ mg of IV morphine}} \quad \text{or} \quad \frac{30}{120} = \frac{10}{X}$$

so   30X = 1200   or   X = 1200/30
                        X = 40 mg IV morphine in 24 hours

- Consider dose reduction because of cross tolerance (No dose reduction for cross tolerance is needed because this is the same opioid, just a different route!).
- Continuous hourly dose is 40 mg/24 hours = **1.66 mg/hour**

Changing the Opioid with the Same Route of Administration

- A patient is being titrated for pain control with Lortab 5/500 and is controlled with 1 Lortab given every 4 hours around the clock. The family wants him to be switched to something he can take less often that has the same pain control effect. How much MS Contin will be needed?

- Figure out the 24-hour dose of hydrocodone: 5 mg every 4 hours (6 times per day) = 5 mg × 6, or 30 mg per 24 hours.

- Look up the equianalgesic value of hydrocodone: 30 mg of oral hydrocodone is the same as 30 mg of oral morphine.

- Do the math. They are the same potency, one to one, so no other calculations are needed. This one is easy!

- Consider cross tolerance: These are different opioids, so cross tolerance could apply and the dose would be reduced by 50%. However, clinically, at this low dose, cross tolerance would probably not be a major concern. As always the patient should be reassessed frequently and clinical judgment applied.

- This patient needs 30 mg of oral morphine per 24 hours; 30 mg twice a day = **MS Contin 15 mg 2 times/day**.

Changing the Opioid and the Route of Administration

- A cancer patient is on MS Contin, 200 mg twice per day for pain, plus Roxanol, 20 mg five times per day, for breakthrough pain. The hospice wants to switch her to a continuous hydrophone (Dilaudid) pump that delivers the opioid IV. What will the hourly rate be?

  - Figure the 24-hour dose of oral morphine: 200 mg MS Contin × 2 doses/day = 400 mg in 24 hours + 20 mg Roxanol × 5 per day = 100 mg, or a total of 500 mg oral morphine daily.

  - Look up the equianalgesic dose between morphine and hydromorphone: 30 mg of oral morphine = 7.5 mg of oral hydromorphone.

  - Do the math:

$$\frac{30 \text{ mg oral morphine}}{500 \text{ mg oral morphine}} = \frac{7.5 \text{ mg oral hydromorphone}}{X \text{ mg of oral hydromorphone}}$$
$$\frac{30}{500} = \frac{7.5}{X}$$
$$30X = 7.5(500) = 3750$$
$$X = 3750/30 = 125$$

  - So the patient needs 125 mg of *oral* hydromorphone in 24 hours. We want to give it IV!

  - Look up the equianalgesic conversion between oral hydromorphone and IV hydromorphone: 7.5 mg PO = 1.5 mg IV.

  - Do the math again:

$$\frac{7.5 \text{ mg oral hydromorphone}}{125 \text{ mg oral hydromorphone}} = \frac{1.5 \text{ mg of IV hydromorphone}}{X \text{ mg of IV}}$$
$$\frac{7.5}{125} = \frac{1.5}{X}$$
$$7.5X = 1.5(125) = 187.5$$
$$X = 187.5/7.5 = 25 \text{mg of IV hydromorphone in}$$
24 hours or a continuous rate of approximately 1 mg per hour.

  - Consider cross tolerance.

- **Reduce the dose by 50%** initially to avoid cross tolerance (less if pain poorly controlled, more if pain is well controlled). These are different opioids, and at this high dose, cross tolerance of side effects is a real possibility. Assess the patient frequently, however, and be ready to escalate the dose as needed (see Chapter 68 on opioid dose escalation).

- The correct dose will be **0.5 mg per hour of hydromorphone by continuous IV pump**.

- **Shortcuts**

  Once the calculations become familiar, you will notice a few shortcuts:

- **Oral morphine to IV morphine: Divide by 3** (30 mg PO = 10 mg IV) or multiply IV × 3 to get the oral dose! (10 mg IV = 30 mg PO).

- **Oral morphine** and **hydrocodone** have **similar doses**. (Most experts now think that oxycodone is 1.5 times stronger than oral morphine! Older charts, however, place oxycodone as equal to oral morphine.)

- **Oral hydromorphone** (Dilaudid) is **four times** as potent as **oral morphine**. To convert from oral morphine, divide by 4 to get the Dilaudid dose; or multiply the Dilaudid dose by 4 to get the oral morphine dose.

- **IV hydromorphone** (Dilaudid) is **20 times** more potent than oral morphine.

- The conversion from **oral morphine to fentanyl** patch (Duragesic) calculates out to half the 24-hour oral morphine dose, in micrograms rather than milligrams. Simply **divide by 2** and change the milligrams to micrograms (100 mg oral morphine per day = 50 µg fentanyl patch).

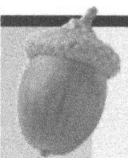

Converting One Opioid to Another (Equianalgesic Dosing)
IN A NUTSHELL

Opioids are unique in that they have equal analgesic effects if given in appropriate doses and routes of administration.

Equianalgesic values are a guide. Use your clinical judgment because each patient is different.

Cross tolerance of side effects is possible when switching opioids, particularly at higher doses.

Calculating equianalgesic doses is simple once mastered:

Figure the 24-hour dose of the opioid.

Convert that dose to oral morphine.

Look up the equianalgesic dose.

Do the math in ratios.

Consider a 50% dose reduction because of cross tolerance.

Remember, these are guidelines. Clinical judgment is still imperative!

- **Comment**

At first, doing the preceding calculations seems more difficult than simply looking at a chart where all the doses are precalculated for dose conversions. However, those charts are very voluminous and complex with so many opioids now being used. It is easy to make an error using that type of chart.

Learning to calculate the doses from equianalgesic values affirms an understanding of opioid dosing, and errors are much less likely. For example, if you know that IV morphine is three times stronger than PO, a mistake would easily be recognized if the dose goes up when converting from PO to IV. **Thinking and understanding** is always better than depending on values from precalculated dose conversion charts.

REFERENCES

1. Gordon DB, Stevenson KK, Griffie J, et al. Opioid equianalgesic calculations. J Palliat Med. 1999;2:209–218.
2. Knight SJ, von Gunten C. *Endlink—Resource for End of Life Care*. National Cancer Institute & Department of Veterans Affairs. Health Services Research and Development Service Career Development Award. Available at: http://endlink.lurie.northwestern.edu/pain_management/part_two.cfm#Opioid%20Cross-Tolerance. Accessed on April 14, 2006.
3. Kansas Foundation for Medical Care; Centers for Medicare & Medicaid Services. *Pain Management Principles and Medications Pocket Guide for the Geriatric Individual*. Publication 7SOW-KS-NHQI-05–35. Washington, DC: U.S. Department of Health and Human Services; 2005.
4. Weissman DE. *Improving End-of-Life Care: A Faculty Development Course Book for Medical Educators*. Milwaukee: The Medical College of Wisconsin; 2000.

CHAPTER 68

Opioid Dose Escalation

"Start low and go slow" is the motto for most pain medications. Yet if you are the patient in pain, you want control as soon as possible. Patients **vary** a great deal in the **dose of opioids** that they need for pain relief. Therefore, **escalation** of the opioid dose should be done until either the pain is controlled or intolerable side effects develop, which cannot be managed by simple interventions (1).

STARTING DOSE

The World Health Organization (WHO) **analgesic ladder** should be followed (2). Most patients have tried step 1 analgesics (acetaminophen, ibuprofen, etc.) before seeing a health professional. If the step 2 opioid/nonopioid combinations have not been tried, that is a good starting point. The **medication chosen** and the **dose** depend on the **severity of the pain**: hydrocodone/acetaminophen (Lortab), 2.5/500 mg for mild pain, up to oxycodone/acetaminophen (Percocet), 10/325 mg every 4 hours for more significant pain. If the combinations are not controlling the pain, then starting with a morphine equivalent (step 3) of about 10 mg every 4 hours is reasonable and safe.

If the patient is already taking more than that, the starting dose could be higher. For example, a patient who is taking two Lortab, 10/500 each dose, is already getting an equivalent of 20 mg of oral morphine with each dose (20 mg of hydrocodone = 20 mg of oral morphine (see Chapter 67 on equianalgesic dosing).

DOSE ESCALATION

The analgesic response to opioids increases in a linearly fashion, whereas the dose is logarithmic. This means that the **dose should be increased by a percentage** rather than by milligrams. For example, increasing an IV rate of morphine from 1 mg per hour to 2 mg per hour is a 100% increase, which is significant. However, increasing from 5 mg to 6 mg per hour is only a 20% increase and probably will not have much effect on the analgesia (3).

An easy illustration is to think of this as using Lasix. If 40 mg is not working, most clinicians do not increase the dose to 42 mg or 45 mg! They go directly to 80 mg, or a

100% increase! Yet they may increase the morphine drip from 10 to 11 mg, only a 10% increase, which does not make pharmacological sense.

These are **reasonable guidelines** that are both safe and clinically effective (4):

- For **mild pain** (1–3/10), increase the dose by **25%**.
- For **moderate** to severe pain (4–6/10), increase the dose by **25% to 50%**.
- For **severe pain** (7–10/10), increase the dose by **50% to 100%**.

FREQUENCY OF DOSE ESCALATION

The **rate** of dose titration should depend on the **severity of the pain** and the **response of the titration**. The patient must be **assessed** before each dose escalation. Advise the patient that the pain level will most likely not become "0," but we are attempting to balance analgesia with side effects. Dose escalation can safely be done as follows:

- **IV dosing**: every **15 to 30 minutes** until pain is relieved and oral dosing can be initiated.
- **Short-acting oral opioids** (hydrocodone, oxycodone, morphine): every **2 to 4 hours**.
- Long-acting or **sustained-release opioids** (MS Contin, OxyContin, etc.): every **24 hours**. However short-acting opioids can be given for **breakthrough (rescue)** as often as **every hour** (dose at 10% to 20% of the total 24-hour dose—see "Breakthrough Dose" later) and the total 24-hour dose reviewed daily.
- **Transdermal** fentanyl (Duragesic patch): every **72 hours**, but rescue medications are recommended as mentioned earlier.

PRINCIPLES OF TITRATION

The **goal** is to get the **pain under control** and to do it as **quickly** as possible without creating significant side effects. But **each patient is different**! There is **no ceiling** dose for opioids, and absolute dose is immaterial as long as there is a **balance between analgesia and side effects**. Sometimes the total doses used in palliative medicine are impressive. It is not uncommon in certain cancer pain patients for them to take in excess of 2,000 mg of morphine in 24 hours, with good pain control and no side effects.

A couple of proven methods to **initiate pain control** when pain is **severe** and out of control include the following:

- Titrate IV morphine every 30 minutes until pain relief is observed; then begin an oral regimen based on the total amount of IV morphine required in 24 hours (see Chapter 67).
- Begin a scheduled dose of immediate-release morphine every 4 hours and the same dose every 1 hour as needed for breakthrough pain. Then in 24 hours calculate the total dose of morphine required, and increase the scheduled dose to meet that requirement. Once the 24-hour dose is known, the morphine can be switched to long-acting dosage (4).

BREAKTHROUGH (RESCUE) DOSE

Once titration is accomplished and steady state is achieved with either scheduled immediate-release opioid or with sustained-release medication, a breakthrough or rescue dose should be available:

- Recommended breakthrough dose is **10% to 20%** of the **total 24-hour dose**, offered (4):
  - **Orally** every **1 hour** as needed
  - **IM or SC** every **30 min** as needed
  - **IV** every **10 to 15 minutes** as needed

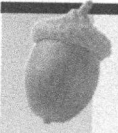

Opioid Dose Escalation
IN A NUTSHELL

Dose escalation is based on the patient's report of uncontrolled pain and assessment, and it is done by **percentage** of the present dose (see Figure 10).

Breakthrough or rescue doses should be calculated as **10% to 20% of the total 24-hour dose** and be available **every hour for PO, every 30 minutes IM or SC, and every 10 to 15 minutes IV, as needed**.

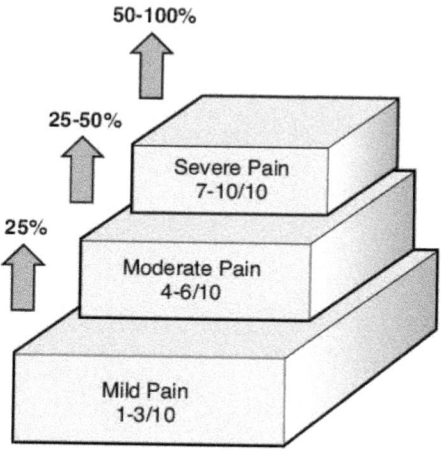

FIGURE 10 •

REFERENCES

1. Hanks G, Cherry, NI, Fulton M. Opioid analgesic therapy. In: Doyle D, Hanks G, Cherny NI, et al., eds. *Oxford Textbook of Palliative Medicine*. 3rd ed. New York: Oxford University Press; 2004:330.
2. World Health Organization. *WHO Ladder: Cancer Pain Relief and Palliative Care*. Technical Report Series 804. Geneva: Author; 1990.

3. Weissman DE, Ambuel B. *Improving End-of-Life Care: A Resource Guide for Physician Education.* Milwaukee: The Medical College of Wisconsin; 1999.
4. Ferris FD, von Gunten CF, Emanuel LL Ensuring competency in end-of-life care: controlling symptoms BMC Palliat Care. 2002;1:5. Published online before print, July 30, 2002.

CHAPTER 69

Managing Opioid Side Effects

Patient compliance generally improves when the clinician takes time to educate patients and their families about the possible side effects of opioids (1). Reassurance should be given that side effects are treatable and, with the exception of constipation, other side effects will **improve in a few days** even without treatment. Side effects do *not* mean the patient is **allergic** to morphine.

COMMON ADVERSE SIDE EFFECTS

Remember that every patient is different, and patients can exhibit almost any side effect imaginable. However, these are the **common side effects** of opioids:

- Constipation—nearly 100%.
- Nausea and/or vomiting—10% to 40%
- Sedation/drowsiness
- Confusion
- Hallucinations
- Pruritus
- Urinary retention—sometimes secondary to constipation-related impaction
- Myoclonic jerks
- Respiratory depression

STRATEGIES FOR MANAGING OPIOID SIDE EFFECTS

Most side effects are **specific** to the type of **opioid** being used and are **dose related**. There are four general ways that opioid side effects can be managed:

1. **Stop or decrease the dose of the opioid**. Slow reduction of the dose can be attempted. However, if pain relief is good and it increases when the dose is reduced, it may be in the patient's best interest to try another strategy. Other possible treatments,

such as radiation to reduce tumor size, nerve blocks, or NSAIDs for bone pain, among others, may reduce the need for as much opioid, thus reducing side effects.

2. **Change the route or type of administration**. For example, sustained-release morphine may be more GI friendly than immediate-release types, particularly on an empty stomach. Perhaps subcutaneous or continuous IV administration (avoiding the GI tract) may be better tolerated.

3. **Switching the opioid**. The reduction of side effects gained by switching from one opioid to another of equal dosage remains clinically controversial (2), but anecdotally it often works. Improvements in cognitive impairment, sedation, and hallucinations are the side effects most often reported to have benefited by this strategy.

4. **Specific therapy to treat the side effects**. This strategy is commonly used and effective. However, no studies have really evaluated the toxicity of this approach over time (3). Adding medications, particularly in the elderly, is always worrisome and may produce side effects of their own. Once again, goals must be considered. In palliative care, pain relief often overshadows other more long-range concerns. Of course, the patient has the option to simply tolerate the side effects if the opioid is effective and the side effects not too severe. Table 10 lists the commonly used **medical treatments**.

TABLE 10

Medical Treatment of Opioid Side Effects (4,5)

Side Effect	Treatment
Constipation	**Senna and docusate sodium (Senokot-S)**: 2 tablets hs and titrate; maximum, 4 tablets bid. **Milk of magnesia**: 30 mL orally and titrate. **Sorbitol**: 15–30 mL PO bid–qid. **Bisacodyl** (Dulcolax): 1–4 tablets bid (more than one laxative may be needed).
Nausea/Vomiting	**Rule out** other causes. **Prochlorperazine** (Compazine): 5–10 mg q6h PO; 25-mg suppositories q12h. **Metoclopramide** (Reglan): 5–10 mg q6h. **Scopolamine** patch: q72h.
Sedation	Wait for sedation to clear. **Methylphenidate** (Ritalin): 2.5–5 mg in AM; repeat at midday if needed. **Dextroamphetamine**: 2.5–5 mg AM and repeat at midday if needed.
Confusion/Hallucinations or delirium	Exclude other causes: sepsis, metabolic imbalance, CNS tumor. **Haloperidol** (Haldol): 5–1 mg PO q6h prn.
Pruritus	Loratadine (Claritin): 10 mg daily PO. Diphenhydramine (Benadryl): 25 mg q6h prn (sedation common). Hydroxyzine (Atarax, Vistaril): 25–100 mg q6–8h prn.
Urinary retention	Catheterization. Tamsulosin (Flomax): 4 mg daily.

Side Effect	Treatment
Myoclonic jerks	Decrease dose or switch opioid. Benzodiazepine of choice: Clonazepam (Klonopin), 0.5 mg tid. Continuous midazolam (Versed) allows rapid titration. Dantrolene (Dantrium): 25 mg daily and titrate to 50–100 mg daily—no sedation.
Respiratory depression	Assess cause. Naloxone (Narcan) to reverse opioid (see Chapter 76).

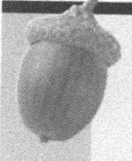

Managing Opioid Side Effects
IN A NUTSHELL

Most opioid side effects, except constipation, improve over time.

Patient education concerning side effects improves patient compliancy.

Common side effects include constipation, nausea/vomiting, sedation, changes in level of consciousness, and pruritus. Other side effects are rare.

Side effects are drug and dose specific.

Treatment options include the following:

Stop or decrease opioid.

Change route of administration.

Switch opioid.

Treat the specific side effect.

Treat the side effects aggressively if the pain is well controlled.

Be aware of side effects from the medications treating the side effects!

REFERENCES

1. Storey P, Knight CF. Assessment and Treatment of Pain in the Terminally Ill. UNIPAC Three. *Hospice/Palliative Care Training for Physicians.* 2nd ed. Glenview, Ill: American Academy of Hospice and Palliative Medicine; 2003:35.
2. Fallon M. Opioid rotation: does it have a role? Palliat Med. 1997;11:177–178.
3. Hanks G, Cherry, NI, Fulton M. Opioid analgesic therapy. In: Doyle D, Hanks G, Cherny NI, et al., eds. *Oxford Textbook of Palliative Medicine.* 3rd ed. New York: Oxford University Press; 2004:316–341.
4. Pain Management Partnership. *Analgesic Reference Guide.* Kansas City: University of Kansas School of Medicine; 2005:KS5.
5. Whitecar PS, Jonas AP, Clasen ME. Managing pain in the dying patient. Am Fam Physician. 2000;61:755–764.

CHAPTER 70

Opioid Withdrawal

Physical dependence is a **normal and predictable** neurophysiological response of patients who take opioids regularly for more than 1 to 2 weeks (1). This characteristic does **not equate with addiction** (2) (see Chapter 63). Although this effect is not as great as once thought in patients taking appropriate pain medications, it must be considered if the opioid is abruptly stopped or if naloxone is given to neutralize the opioid.

SYMPTOMS

Withdrawal or "abstinence syndrome" may be seen as soon as 6 to 12 hours after stopping short-acting opioids (hydrocodone, morphine, hydromorphone, oxycodone) and peak at 24 to 72 hours. In long-acting opioids (methadone, MS Contin, OxyContin, transdermal fentanyl), withdrawal may not start until 24 hours or more after discontinuation. Withdrawal from the **long-acting** medications is usually of **milder intensity** because of the slower clearance from the body.

Other important clinical signs and symptoms commonly encountered include the following:

- Mildest form: **flulike symptoms**.
- Anxiety, irritability, yawning, chills, hot flashes, sweating, joint pain, lacrimation, rhinorrhea, insomnia, nausea, vomiting, abdominal cramps, diarrhea, hypertension, tachycardia, myalgias, piloerection, and dilated pupils.
- Unlike withdrawal from alcohol or benzodiazepines, **opioid withdrawal is not life threatening** (3).

PREVENTION

Opioid withdrawal or abstinence syndrome can be avoided by **gradually tapering** opioids rather than abruptly stopping them. One recommended schedule of withdrawing opioids is as follows (4):

- Give half the previous dose for the first 2 days.
- Then reduce the dose by 25% every 2 days.
- When the dose reaches an equivalent of 30 mg per day or PO morphine (see Chapter 67), give that dose for 2 days and then discontinue.

An **alternative recommendation** (3):

- Reduce the dose 25% every 2 days, and assess the patient frequently.

TREATMENT

If for some reason a tapering dose cannot be given or the patient cannot simply be given a dose of opioid, the following can be done to **treat autonomic hyperactivity**:

- Clonidine (Catapres), 0.1–0.2 mg PO every 4 to 6 hours as needed or by transdermal patch (Catapres TTS 1), 0.1 mg every 7 days.
- Clonidine will not treat insomnia and may cause hypotension.

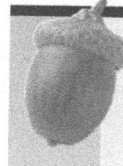

Opioid Withdrawal
IN A NUTSHELL

Physical dependence does **not** equate with psychological **addiction**. Slow **tapering** of the opioid dose should be done on any patient who has taken opioids regularly for 2 weeks or more.

Taper the dose:

Half the dose for the first 2 days; then reduce 25% every 2 days until at 30 mg per day of oral morphine equivalent; give 30 mg for 2 days and then stop.

Decrease dose by 25% every 2 days.

Autonomic hyperactivity can be treated with clonidine, 0.1–0.2 mg PO every 4 to 6 hours, or transdermal patch, 0.1 mg every 7 days.

REFERENCES

1. Sees KL, Clark HW. Opioid use in the treatment of chronic pain: assessment of addiction. J Pain Symptom Manage. 1993;8:257–264.
2. Portenoy RK, Payne R. Acute and chronic pain. In: Lowinson JH, Ruiz P, Millman RB, eds. *Substance Abuse: A Comprehensive Textbook.* 2nd ed. Baltimore: Williams & Wilkins; 1992:691–721.
3. Gordon D, Dahl J. Opioid withdrawal. *Fast Fact and Concepts #95.* Milwaukee: The Medical College of Wisconsin; 2002. Available at: http://www.eperc.mcw.edu/fastFact/ff_95.htm. Accessed April 30, 2006.
4. American Pain Society. *Principles of Analgesic Use in the Treatment of Acute Pain and Chronic Cancer Pain: A Concise Guide to Medical Practice.* Skokie, Ill: Author; 1992.

Morphine

Morphine is a potent μ agonist that has been used for over 200 years to control pain. The World Health Organization has placed oral morphine on the Essential Drug List. Preparations are available for oral, rectal, parenteral, and intraspinal administration (1).

INDICATIONS

Moderate to severe pain:

- Somatic pain
- Visceral pain
- Neuropathic pain (less effective)

SPECIFIC INFORMATION

Table 11 best describes the various forms of morphine, the peak activity (time after which another dose may be given if there is insufficient effect from the previous dose or doses), common durations of analgesia, special precautions, and comments. The **equianalgesic dosing** for morphine is 30 mg oral (or rectal) equals 10 mg parenteral (IV, SC, or IM). Notice the dose is the same for all parenteral administration; however, the time of onset will be faster if given IV. Medication choice, route of administration, and dosing intervals should all be determined by **patient assessment**. Dosing should be decreased in the frail elderly and in patients with known liver disease or renal failure.

SIDE EFFECTS

Many common side effects of morphine administration can be **avoided by proper titration**. Side effects do *not* mean the patient is allergic to morphine. Other than constipation, other side effects will **improve in a few days**. However, if pain relief

TABLE 11

Morphine (2)

Preparation	Doses	Peak	Duration	Precautions	Comments
Immediate Release					
MSIR	15 mg; 30 mg	1 hr	4 hr	Elderly more sensitive to metabolites.	Start low and titrate to comfort; begin bowel program.
Oral Liquid					
MSIR Liquid	2 mg/mL; 4 mg/mL	<1 hr	4 hr	Same.	Same.
Roxanol Concentrate	20 mg/mL	<1 hr	4 hr	Same.	Roxanol-T is orange colored and has a pleasant fruit taste; Roxanol is clear and does not taste good.
Suppository					
Rectal Morphine Sulfate (RMS)	5, 10, 20, 30 mg	1 hr	4 hr	Same.	Same.
Sustained-Release Tablets					
MS Contin	15, 30, 60, 100, 200 mg	3–6 hr	8–12 hr	Escalate doses slowly; need immediate-release opioids for breakthrough pain.	**Do not cut or crush tablets**.
Kadian	20, 30, 50, 60, 100 mg	3–6 hr	24 hr	Same.	Capsule may be opened and poured down a nasogastric (NG) tube.
Oramorph SR	15, 30, 60, 100 mg	3–6 hr	8–12 hr	Same.	Same as MS Contin.
Avinza	30, 60, 90, 120 mg	3–6 hr	24 hr	Same.	Same as MS Contin.
Parenteral Morphine					
	Up to 20 mg/mL	Immediate	4 hr	May cause systemic vasodilation and purities secondary to histamine release.	

is needed, it is better to continue the morphine and **aggressively treat the side effects**, which include the following:

• **Nausea and vomiting**: Occurs in 10% to 40% of patients when first taking morphine (3). Prochlorperazine (Compazine) usually works well to control symptoms. Usually the antiemetic can be phased out after several days.

• **Sedation, drowsiness, and somnolence**: Frequent at the beginning of therapy but usually clears in 2 to 5 days. Restorative sleep is common, where the patient has not been able to sleep well because of pain. Once the pain is relieved the patient may sleep for long periods of time. This is not an undesirable side effect.

• **Pruritus**: Caused by histamine release; usually controlled with diphenhydramine (Benadryl) or hydroxyzine (Atarax, Vistaril).

CONSTIPATION

Count on it, and start treatment when the morphine is started.

> "The finger that holds the pen to write the order for morphine must hold the pen to write for the laxative, or that finger will be used to disimpact the patient."

A stimulant laxative is usually needed. Stool softeners alone are generally not effective. Use Senna (Senokot) or bisacodyl (Dulcolax). Start once per day and titrate if needed. Sorbitol, 15 to 30 mL, can be added, if needed, and titrated.

> **Both a musher and a pusher are needed** (softener plus stimulant).

OVERDOSE

Overdose is rare if appropriate titration procedures are followed. It can occur, however, particularly in the frail elderly. Treatment is to hold the morphine and wait for the drug to wear off. Naloxone (Narcan) is seldom needed but can reverse the effects of the morphine. Be suspicious of overdose in these situations:

• Level of consciousness and respiratory rate both decrease concomitantly, especially if respirations are less than 6 per minute.

• Other signs are present, including myoclonic twitching, constricted pupils, cold or clammy skin, and skeletal muscle flaccidity.

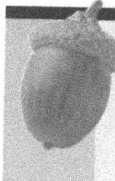

Morphine
IN A NUTSHELL

Morphine is **effective and safe** for treating moderate to severe pain. Proper pain **assessment** should be done to determine administration route and dosage.

Prescribe medication in a way that makes **pharmacological sense**—in relation to onset and duration.

Reassess the patient and titrate morphine to analgesic response. **Start low** and **go slow** in the frail elderly and in patients with liver disease or renal failure.

Treat side effects aggressively—prochlorperazine (Compazine) for nausea and vomiting. Side effects, except constipation, usually resolve in 2 to 5 days.

Anticipate constipation and start a bowel regimen early. Stool softeners (docusate/Colace, etc.) are not enough; use a **stimulant such as Senna**.

Overdose is rare if appropriately dosed, but watch for a combination of decreased level of consciousness, respiratory rate less than 6, constricted pupils, cold clammy skin, and myoclonic twitching.

REFERENCES

1. Hanks G, Cherry, NI, Fulton M. Opioid analgesic therapy. In: Doyle D, Hanks G, Cherny NI, et al., eds. *Oxford Textbook of Palliative Medicine*. 3rd ed. New York: Oxford University Press, 2004:316–341.
2. Kansas Foundation for Medical Care (KFMC) Inc. *Pain Management Principles and Medications Pocket Guide for the Geriatric Individual*. Topeka, Kan: Under contract for the Centers for Medicare & Medicaid Services, an agency of the U.S. Department of Health and Human Services; 2005. Pub. no. 7SOW-KS-NHQI-05–35. Revised July 2005.
3. Storey P, Knight CF. Assessment and Treatment of Pain in the Terminally Ill. UNIPAC Three, *Hospice/Palliative Care Training for Physicians*. 2nd ed. Glenview, Ill: American Academy of Hospice and Palliative Medicine 2003:39.

CHAPTER 72

Hydrocodone for Pain

Hydrocodone is an orally active step 2 opioid analgesic, used for **moderate to moderately severe pain**. Hydrocodone is available only in **combination with acetaminophen or ibuprofen**. These combinations are the dose-limiting factors because there is no ceiling dose on the hydrocodone itself. Combinations are marketed in both **oral tablet and liquid form**, in a variety of dosages.

Hydrocodone combinations are frequently used for breakthrough pain on an as needed basis. For chronic pain it must be given on a regular schedule because of its short half-life. For specific products and dosages, see Table 12.

The side effects are similar to side effects for morphine (see Chapter 71).

TABLE 12

Specific Products and Dosages of Hydrocodone (1,2)

Preparation	Doses	Peak	Duration	Precautions	Comments
Hydrocodone/ acetaminophen tablets				Limit daily acetaminophen dose to 4 g; less in elderly (3 g) or in liver disease; toxicity of hydrocodone similar to morphine.	Start bowel program early; start low and titrate.
Lorcet	10/650 mg	1 hr	4 hr	Same.	
Lorcet HD	5/500 mg	1 hr	4 hr	Same.	
Lorcet Plus	7.5/650 mg	1 hr	4 hr	Same.	
Lortab	2.5/500 mg	1 hr	4 hr	Same.	
	5/500 mg				
	7.5/500 mg				
	10/500 mg				

Preparation	Doses	Peak	Duration	Precautions	Comments
Maxidone	10/750 mg	1 hr	4 hr	Same.	
Norco	5/325 mg	1 hr	4 hr	Same.	
	7.5/325 mg				
	10/325 mg				
Vicodin	5/500 mg	1 hr	4 hr	Same.	
Vicodin ES	7.5/750	1 hr	4 hr	Same.	
Vicodin HP	10/650 mg	1 hr	4 hr	Same.	
Hydrocodone/ acetaminophen liquid					
Lortab Elixir	7.5/500 mg per 15 mL	1 hr	4 hr	Same.	
Hydrocodone/ ibuprofen tablets				Watch for side effects (mostly gastrointestinal) of ibuprofen; toxicity of hydrocodone similar to morphine.	Maximum daily dose limited by ibuprofen; start bowel program early; start low and titrate.
Vicoprofen	7.5/200 mg	1 hr	4 hr	Same.	As above.
Zydone	5/400 mg	1 hr	4 hr	Same.	As above.
	7.5/400 mg				
	10/400 mg				

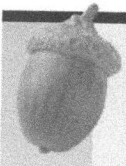

Hydrocodone for Pain
IN A NUTSHELL

Hydrocodone is a step 2 opioid used for **breakthrough pain**, as well as for chronic pain.

Hydrocodone is available only in **combination** with **acetaminophen** or **ibuprofen**. A number of products and doses are obtainable.

The acetaminophen or ibuprofen is the **limiting factor** in dosing hydrocodone.

Side effects are similar to other **opioids**.

REFERENCES

1. Narcotic analgesics. Monthly Prescribing Reference. March 2006;22:288.
2. Kansas Foundation for Medical Care (KFMC) Inc. *Pain Management Principles and Medications Pocket Guide for the Geriatric Individual.* Topeka, Kan: Under contract for the Centers for Medicare & Medicaid Services, an agency of the U.S. Department of Health and Human Services; 2005. Pub no. 7SOW-KS-NHQI-05–35. Revised July 2005.

CHAPTER 73

Oxycodone for Pain

Oxycodone is a synthetic morphine congener that has high oral bioavailability. It has an analgesic potency greater than equal doses of morphine (1). Oxycodone is available in both **immediate-acting tablets** and **liquid sustained-release** formulations and in **combination products**. There is **no ceiling** dose for **oxycodone**, but care must be exercised in using the combination products because the acetaminophen, aspirin, or ibuprofen is the dose-limiting factor.

There has been recent negative press about the **diversion** of OxyContin for illicit drug use outside of legitimate medical practice. However, with proper use in the areas of palliative care, OxyContin remains an **effective long-acting oral analgesic**.

INDICATIONS

- Moderate to severe pain:

SPECIFIC PRODUCTS AND DOSAGES

Oxycodone is available in a number of doses and combination doses. Although there has been some controversy about the equianalgesic potency of oxycodone, most pain guides now consider oxycodone to be more potent than an equal dose of oral morphine in a ratio of 1.5 to 1 (30 mg of oral morphine = 20 mg of oral oxycodone) (2). Equianalgesic values are only meant to be guidelines, so the clinician needs to use clinical judgment, as usual, in calculating doses.

Table 13 lists the **common preparations** of oxycodone.

SIDE EFFECTS

Current data indicate that there is **no significant difference** in side effects for oxycodone as **compared to the other opioids** (4):

- Major side effects include nausea/vomiting, sedation, and constipation (see Chapter 71).

- There is **no increase** in potential **tolerance, physical dependence**, or psychological dependence (**addiction**) over other opioids.

TABLE 13

Common Preparations of Oxycodone

Preparation	Doses	Peak	Duration	Precautions	Comments
Immediate Release					
OxyIR and Roxicodone tablets	5 mg	1 hr	3–4 hr		
OxyFAST liquid	20 mg/mL	1 hr	3–4 hr		
Roxicodone liquid	1 mg/mL and 20 mg/mL	1 hr	3–4 hr		
Combinations					
Oxycodone/ Acetaminophen					
Percocet	2.5/325 5/325 7.5/325 7.5/500 10/325 10/650	1 hr	3–4 hr	Maximum daily dose of combination limited to 4,000 mg of acetaminophen.	**Decrease acetaminophen dose in elderly.**
Roxicet	5/325 5/500	1 hr	3–4 hr	Same.	Same.
Tylox	5/500	1 hr	3–4 hr	Same	Same.
Oxycodone/Aspirin					
Percodan	2.5/325 5/325	1 hr	3–4 hr	Precautions related to aspirin.	
Oxycodone/ibuprofen					
Combunox	5/400	1 hr	3–4 hr	Precautions related to ibuprofen.	Avoid ibuprofen in the elderly; gastrointestinal precautions.
Sustained Release					
OxyContin	10 mg 20 mg 40 mg 80 mg	Possibly 1 hr (3); steady state in 24 hr	8–12 hr	Do not cut or crush tablets; do not use rectally.	More expensive (6–10 times) than controlled-release morphine products; need immediate-release medication for breakthrough pain.

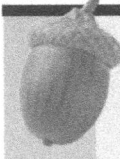

Oxycodone for Pain
IN A NUTSHELL

Oxycodone is **effective** for moderate to severe pain and is available in a number of preparations, including oral tablets, sustained-release tablets, liquid, and a number of combination products (combined with acetaminophen, aspirin, or ibuprofen).

There is **no ceiling dose** for oxycodone; however, the medication used in the **combination products must be watched carefully** (limit acetaminophen dose to less than 4 g in 24 hours—less in liver disease and the elderly).

Analgesic potency is **1.5 times that of morphine**.

Side effects are equal with those of morphine.

OxyContin (sustained release) is more **expensive** than many other opioids.

REFERENCES

1. Kalso E, Vainio A. Morphine and oxycodone hydrochloride in the management of cancer pain. Clin Pharmacol Ther. 1990;47:639–646.
2. Kansas Foundation for Medical Care (KFMC) Inc. *Pain Management Principles and Medications Pocket Guide for the Geriatric Individual.* Topeka, Kan: Under contract for the Centers for Medicare & Medicaid Services, an agency of the U.S. Department of Health and Human Services; 2005. Pub no. 7SOW-KS-NHQI-05–35. Revised July 2005.
3. Hanks G, Cherry, NI, Fulton M. Opioid analgesic therapy. In: Doyle D, Hanks G, Cherny NI, et al., eds. *Oxford Textbook of Palliative Medicine.* 3rd ed. New York: Oxford University Press; 2004:325.
4. Weissman DE. OxyContin. *Fast Facts and Concepts #80.* Milwaukee: The Medical College of Wisconsin; 2002. Available at: http://www.eperc.mcw.edu/fastFact/ff_80.htm. Accessed March 8, 2006.

CHAPTER 74

Methadone for Pain Control

Methadone is a potent opioid agonist that has been available for decades. However, its use is gaining renewed interest in modern palliative care because of its **low cost** and **effectiveness in neuropathic pain** (1). Any clinician with a Schedule II DEA certificate can prescribe methadone for pain, but a special license is needed to use it for treating addiction. **Writing the words "for pain" on the script** helps clarify this difference.

INDICATIONS

Moderate to severe chronic pain:

- Especially effective for visceral and neuropathic pain.

SPECIFIC INFORMATION

Methadone is available in these forms:

- Tablets (Dolophine), 5 mg, 20 mg, 40 mg (hard to find); tablets may be used rectally.
- Liquid (generic methadone), 1 mg, 2 mg, or 10 mg per mL.
- Injectable, 10 mg per mL for IV. IM and SC use is limited because of skin and tissue inflammation.
- There is **no maximum dose** for methadone.

UNIQUE CHARACTERISTICS OF METHADONE

When compared to morphine and the other opioids, methadone has some very unique characteristics that demand special consideration:

- The **half-life** of methadone is **variable and very long,** with a range of over 150 hours. It accumulates with each dose.
- The **analgesic effects** of methadone last only **6 to 12 hours** after steady state is reached.

- The long half-life can lead to **overmedication** with risk of increased sedation and respiratory depression, especially in the frail elderly.
- **Titration**, therefore, must be very slow with dose adjustments done only about once **every 4 to 7 days** (2,3). The rapid titration guidelines used with the other opioids do not apply and can be dangerous.
- Methadone is not a good choice for poorly controlled pain where rapid dose adjustments are needed.
- Methadone has a lack of known metabolites, so **no dose adjustments** are needed for **renal insufficiency**.
- Methadone works better than other opioids on **neuropathic pain**.
- Methadone is metabolized by the **cytochrome P450** enzyme:
  - Methadone levels are **increased by** amitriptyline, ciprofloxacin, diazepam, fluconazole, fluoxetine, erythromycin, metronidazole, propoxyphene, spironolactone, grapefruit juice, and others.
  - Methadone levels **decreased by** rifampin, phenytoin, carbamazepine, and many antiretrovirals.
- Methadone is **inexpensive** and, once titrated properly, **gives good pain control with few side effects** and little euphoria.

DOSING METHADONE

Titrating the correct dose is the most difficult part of using methadone. Patients must be **educated** that they will not experience immediate results. There is also a sigma attached to methadone, and some patients are concerned the clinician will think they are addicted. Therefore, **patient compliance** is crucial in getting good results from methadone.

Once steady state is reached (approximately 5 to 7 days), most patients are well controlled on dosing every 8 to 12 hours; an occasional patient may require dosing every 4 to 8 hours (3).

Converting the dose of **morphine to methadone** has been fraught with **controversy and confusion**. Pain management consultation with someone experienced in using methadone for pain may be appropriate in initially establishing a methadone regimen for a patient. However, the general conversions in Table 14 have been used (4).

TABLE 14

General Guidelines for Converting Morphine to Methadone Dosage

For a 24-hour oral morphine dose of:

- <100 mg — Use 3:1 morphine to methadone
- 101–300 mg — Use 5:1
- 301–600 mg — Use 10:1
- 601–800 mg — Use 12:1
- 801–1,000 mg — Use 15:1
- >1,000 mg — Use 20:1

Note: Other conversion tables are also available.

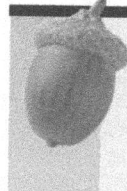

Methadone for Pain Control
IN A NUTSHELL

Methadone is indicated for chronic moderate to severe pain as well as neuropathic pain, but it has a number of **unique characteristics** that make it more difficult to use than morphine.

Methadone has a very **long and variable half-life**, which makes **accumulation** of medication a hazard.

Doses should not be increased faster than every **4 to 7 days**.

No dosage adjustments are needed for **renal insufficiency**.

Cytochrome P450 enzyme is involved in metabolism.

Converting from morphine to methadone requires special protocols.

Write "For Pain" on the script!

REFERENCES

1. Gazelle G, Fine PG. Methadone for the treatment of pain. *Fast Facts and Concepts #75.* Milwaukee: The Medical College of Wisconsin; 2002. Available at: http://www.eperc.mcw.edu/fastFact/ff_75.htm. Accessed April 1, 2006.
2. Bruera E, Sweeney C. Methadone use in cancer patients with pain: A review. J Palliat Med. 2002;5:127–138.
3. Hanks G, Cherry, NI, Fulton M. Opioid analgesic therapy. In: Doyle D, Hanks G, Cherny NI, et al., eds. *Oxford Textbook of Palliative Medicine.* 3rd ed. New York: Oxford University Press; 2004:324–325.
4. Gazelle G, Fine PG. Methadone for pain: no. 75. J Palliat Med. 2004;7:303–304.

CHAPTER 75

Gabapentin (Neurontin) for Pain

Gabapentin (Neurontin) is now widely used for the treatment of chronic neuropathic pain syndromes. A number of controlled clinical studies suggest that gabapentin is superior to placebo in treating neuropathic pain associated with diabetic neuropathy, cancer pain syndromes, pain associated with HIV infection, and others (1).

Tricyclic antidepressants, such as amitriptyline (Elavil), have traditionally been used for neuropathic pain and have been extensively studied. Although amitriptyline shows similar efficacy with gabapentin (2), the side effects (most notably anticholinergic responses of dry mouth, fatigue, headache, and orthostatic hypotension) seem to be much higher, particularly in the elderly patient (3).

SPECIFICS

When considering the use of gabapentin for pain, patients should be thoroughly assessed to determine that they have a neuropathic pain syndrome, consisting of sharp, shooting, lancinating and/or burning pain in a nerve root (radicular) or stocking/glove distribution.

Some of the specific characteristics of gabapentin include the following:

- The exact mechanism and site of action is unknown.
- It is generally well tolerated, with fewer side effects than the tricyclic antidepressants (amitriptyline).
- Blood levels do not require laboratory monitoring.
- There are few drug interactions.
- Gabapentin is available in 100-mg, 300-mg, and 400-mg capsules; 600-mg and 800-mg tablets; and a liquid (250 mg per 5 mL).
- Cost may be a limiting factor for some patients.
- It is easily titrated with a usual effective total daily dose of 900 to 3,600 mg, given in three divided doses per day.

- Adult dosing: Start at low doses of 100 mg daily to 100 mg three times per day and increase 100 to 300 mg every 1 to 3 days until pain is relieved. (A typical schedule could include day 1 and 2—300 mg HS; day 3 and 4—300 mg BID; day 5 and 6—600 mg BID; day 7 and beyond—600 mg TID, etc.) (4). Higher doses may be used.

- Titration should be slower in the elderly or frail patient.

- In renal insufficiency, the dose is reduced (5): creatinine clearance, 30 to 59: maximum dose is 400 to 1,400 mg per day, given twice daily; creatinine clearance, 15 to 29: maximum dose is 200 to 700 mg daily; creatinine clearance <15: maximum dose is 100 to 300 mg once daily.

- Hemodialysis: Maximum dose is 125 to 350 mg only after each dialysis session.

ADVERSE REACTIONS

Slow titration helps prevent common side effects. Side effects seem to resolve within a few days if the dose is held steady. Titration can then begin again when the side effects are tolerable to the patient. Common adverse effects include the following:

- Sedation or somnolence
- Confusion
- Dizziness
- Ataxia or abnormal gait
- Gastrointestinal upset
- Peripheral edema

Gabapentin (Neurontin) for Pain
IN A NUTSHELL

Gabapentin is effective in treating neuropathic pain.

Tricyclic antidepressants are as effective as gabapentin and less expensive, but they have more side effects.

The patient should be assessed and the diagnosis of neuropathic pain presumed before gabapentin is tried.

Typical doses range from 900 mg to 3,600 mg, or more.

Dosage should be titrated.

Side effects generally resolve if titration is slowed.

REFERENCES

1. Corbett CF. Practical management of patients with painful diabetic neuropathy. Diabetes Educ. 2005 Jul-Aug; 31:523–540.
2. Wiffen PJ, McQuay HJ, Edwards JE, et al. Gabapentin for acute and chronic pain. Cochrane Database Syst Rev. 2005;(3):CD005452. Available at: www.cochrane.org/newslett/ NeurologicalNetworkOrangePages12006.pdf.
3. Beers MH. Explicit criteria for determining potentially inappropriate medication use by the elderly [abstract]. Arch Intern Med. 1977;157:1531–1536.
4. Kishore A, King L. Gabapentin for neuropathic pain. *Fast Facts and Concepts # 49.* Milwaukee: The Medical College of Wisconsin. Available at: http://www.eperc.mcw.edu/ fastFact/ff_49.htm. Accessed April 11, 2006.
5. Monthly Prescribing Reference. March 2006;22:282.

CHAPTER 76

Naloxone (Narcan)

Naloxone (Narcan) is a semisynthetic **opioid antagonist** used to **reverse** the effects of any opioid. Ideally it is indicated to reverse dangerous or life-threatening CNS/ respiratory depression induced by opioids. However, **naloxone is often inappropriately used** in the hospital in response to physiologically normal opioid-induced decrease in respiratory rate or mild sedation (1).

INDICATIONS

It is **normal** to have a **decreased respiratory rate** during sleep, especially when taking opioids. In addition, patients who have had untreated pain for some time may experience "**restorative sleep**" (sometimes sleeping for several days) when their pain is finally under control and they can relax. These situations **do not need treatment** with naloxone.

Indications for naloxone in palliative care are few:

- Naloxone is indicated for **significant opioid-induced CNS depression**, the hall-mark being severe change in the level of consciousness.

  - The patient should be very **difficult to arouse or unarousable**. If the patient awakens to verbal stimuli or to a light shake, the diagnosis is sleeping, not opioid overdose.

  - A patient should have **shallow respirations of less than 8 per minute** with **evidence of inadequate ventilation** (e.g., low oxygen saturation or hypotension). Some people may normally breathe 6 to 8 times per minute while asleep. They are still well oxygenated.

  - Remember, patients will have a **predictable sequence of events with opioid overdose**—going from awake to drowsy, to more sedated, to less arousable, to comatose, to respiratory depression, to serious respiratory depression. Patients do not go from awake to dead with appropriate doses without going through these predictable stages.

NOT INDICATED

Naloxone is *not* **indicated** in the following patients:

- **Patients on opioids who are dying**. All dying patients at some point have an altered mentation and respiratory slowing. Administering naloxone in this circumstance may cause the abrupt return of pain and suffering (2).
- **Other opioid side effects**, such as nausea, vomiting, constipation, hives, or multifocal myoclonus. These side effects can be managed otherwise as detailed elsewhere.

USING NALOXONE

If it is believed that the patient truly has significant opioid-induced CNS or respiratory depression, the following treatments should be used:

- **Stop the opioid** administration.
- **Monitor the patient** and **wait** for the effects of the opioid to wear off if possible. This is especially desirable if the peak effect of the last opioid dose has already been reached.
- **Remind the patient to breathe**: "Take a deep breath!" Many patients respond to this.
- Consider placing an endotracheal tube in the comatose patient to prevent aspiration after giving the naloxone (3).
- **Dilute** one ampule of naloxone (0.4 mg) with normal saline to make a total volume of 10 mL. In this dilution, 1 mL = 0.04 mg of naloxone. (1:10 dilution)
- Give **small IV boluses** (1 mL) of the dilute solution every 1 to 2 minutes, titrating to the patient's respiratory rate or mental responsiveness. This **gentle titration** prevents acute opioid withdrawal and return of severe pain. Usually a response is noticed after 2 to 4 mL of the dilute solution is given. Do *not* give the full undiluted ampule at once.
- If the patient does not respond to 2 ampules (0.8 mg) given as described, consider some other cause of the sedation or respiratory depression!
- Remember that the **duration of action for naloxone** is **shorter** than most short-acting opioids, so access the patient frequently because **another dose, or even a constant infusion, may be needed**.
- Completely **reevaluate** the patient before restarting opioids at a lower dose.

ADVERSE EFFECTS

In addition to creating acute withdrawal of the opioid and the rapid return of pain, naloxone has the following adverse effects (4):

- Cardiac arrest/ventricular fibrillation
- Pulmonary edema
- Hypertension/hypotension

- Seizures
- Nausea/vomiting

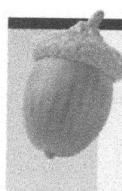

Naloxone (Narcan)
IN A NUTSHELL

Naloxone (Narcan) can be used to **reverse the effects of opioids**.

Naloxone **can precipitate severe withdrawal** and rapid return of pain in patients on appropriate doses of opioids for pain control.

Naloxone should only be used if **strongly indicated** in palliative care patients. Stopping the opioid and waiting for it to clear the body should be considered.

This medication should be administered only in patients where **severe CNS/respiratory depression/hypoventilation** is present.

If indicated, naloxone should be **diluted** in normal saline in a 1:10 ratio and then **titrated 1 mL** at a time IV until the patient responds. If there is no improvement after 2 ampules (0.8 mg) are given, reassess the diagnosis.

REFERENCES

1. Dunwoody CJ, Arnold R. Using naloxone. *Fast Facts and Concepts #39*. Milwaukee: The Medical College of Wisconsin; 2002. Available at: http://www.eperc.mcw.edu/fastFact/ff_39.htm. Accessed April 22, 2006.
2. Foley K. A 44-year-old woman with severe pain at the end of life. JAMA. 1999; 281: 1937–1945.
3. Hanks G, Cherry, NI, Fulton M. Opioid analgesic therapy. In: Doyle D, Hanks G, Cherny NI, et al., eds. *Oxford Textbook of Palliative Medicine*. 3rd ed. New York: Oxford University Press; 2004:335.
4. Fang E., ed. *Epocrates Rx*, Version 7.02. Updated October 22, 2005.

CHAPTER 77

Meperidine (Demerol): Not Recommended for Pain

Meperidine is a **weak synthetic opioid** with **adverse effects** that limits its usefulness in palliative care (1). Until recently, meperidine was commonly used for postoperative pain, and its usage carried over into using it for other types of pain. However, a number of **problems** with meperidine have resulted in it no longer being recommended for chronic or acute pain (2).

WHAT ARE THE PROBLEMS WITH MEPERIDINE (DEMEROL)?

These properties of meperidine make it less desirable for treating pain than a number of other medications:

- Very **weak potency**: 75 to 100 mg of meperidine equals 10 mg parenteral morphine; 300 mg of meperidine equals 30 mg of oral morphine.
- **Short duration** of action: Only 2.5 to 3.5 hours.
- **Toxic metabolites**: Accumulation of normeperidine, which has twice the convulsant activity and half the analgesic activity as the parent compound (3). Common adverse reactions include the following:
  - CNS excitation
  - Myoclonus
  - Delirium
  - Seizures

MYTHS

All the national pain management *Clinical Practice Guidelines* published since 1990 have indicated that meperidine (Demerol) is **not recommended** for treating chronic pain. There are **no good data** to support the previous thoughts that meperidine has an advantage in the treatment of these situations:

- Sickle cell pain (4)
- Pain from pancreatitis (5)
- Pain associated with biliary colic

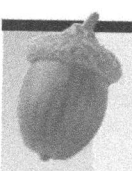

Meperidine (Demerol)
IN A NUTSHELL

With the availability of so many other good medications, there is little rationale for using meperidine for pain treatment.

REFERENCES

1. Hanks G, Cherry, NI, Fulton M. Opioid analgesic therapy. In: Doyle D, Hanks G, Cherny NI, et al., eds. *Oxford Textbook of Palliative Medicine*. 3rd ed. New York: Oxford University Press; 2004:316–341.
2. Weissman DE. Meperidine for pain: what's all the fuss? *Fast Facts and Concepts #71*. 2002 Milwaukee: The Medical College of Wisconsin; 2002. Available at: http://www.eperc.mcw.edu/fastFact/ff_71.htm. Accessed March 27, 2006.
3. Simopoulos TT, Smith HS, Peeters-Asdourian, et al. Use of meperidine in patient-controlled analgesia and the development of a normeperidine toxic reaction. Arch Surg. 2002;137:84–88.
4. *Guideline for the Management of Acute and Chronic Pain in Sickle Cell Disease*. Glenview, Ill: American Pain Society; 1999.
5. Isenhower HL, Mueller BA. Selection of narcotic analgesics for pain associated with pancreatitis. Am J Health Syst Pharm 1998;55:480–486.

CHAPTER 78

Propoxyphene (Darvon, Darvocet)

Propoxyphene (Darvon, Darvocet) is **not recommended** for routine treatment of acute or chronic pain (1). However, it continues to be prescribed frequently (2), probably because of the **false assumption** that it is somehow more potent than acetaminophen but does not have the narcotic stigma of the opioids.

PROBLEMS WITH PROPOXYPHENE

Many clinical trials have shown that propoxyphene has an **analgesic effect equal with placebo** (3). When combined with acetaminophen, propoxyphene has an analgesic effect approximately equal to that of acetaminophen or aspirin (4). Yet, when compared with placebo, acetaminophen, or aspirin, propoxyphene has a **significant increase in side effects**, including the following (5):

- Poor efficacy
- CNS depression/sedation
- Addictive potential
- Adjustment required for liver and renal dosing
- Nausea/vomiting
- Dizziness
- Seizures

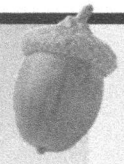

Propoxyphene (Darvon, Darvocet)
IN A NUTSHELL

Propoxyphene provides minimal if any additional analgesia to acetaminophen alone but adds significant adverse effects. Therefore it is **not recommended**.

REFERENCES

1. Zhan C, Sangl J, Bierman AS, et al. Potentially inappropriate medication use in the community dwelling elderly—findings from the 1996 medical expenditure panel survey. JAMA. 2001;286:2823–2829.
2. Kamal-Bahl S, Stuart BC, Beers MH. Am J Geriatr Pharmacother. 2005;3:186–195.
3. LiWan Po A, Zhang WY. Systematic overview of co-proxamol to assess analgesic effects of addition of dextropropoxyphene to paracetamol. BMJ 1997;315:1565–1571.
4. Miller RR. Propoxyphene: a review. Am J Hosp Pharm. 1977;34:413–423.
5. Sachs CJ. Oral analgesics for acute nonspecific pain. Am Fam Physician. 2005;71:913–918.

CHAPTER 79

Blocks

Occasionally **pain cannot be adequately controlled** with the systemic medications described on the WHO ladder. Then the analgesic ladder must be extended to a **fourth level**, which involves **interventional anesthetic nerve blocks** (1). These interventions should most often be performed by an anesthesiologist or other trained pain specialist.

The use of anesthetic nerve block techniques for pain control does not preclude the use of systemic analgesics. Most often, combinations of systemic medications and interventional nerve blocks provide the most effective relief.

INDICATIONS

In the last decade, there has been tremendous **expansion of nerve block techniques**, including radiofrequency neural ablation and injection of botulinum toxin. A number of patient and disease factors may limit the effectiveness of systemic analgesics, providing an indication for interventional nerve blocks (2):

- Neuropathic pain not responding to other therapy
- Resistant cancer pain, such as invasion of cancer into nerve tissue (e.g., a Pancoast tumor invading the brachial plexus)
- Pain that fluctuates markedly in intensity
- Patient that has severe adverse effects (uncontrollable) to systemic medications.
- **Any intractable pain** not controlled by appropriate doses of systemic analgesics or other pain relief methods

TYPES OF BLOCKS

With proper technique, almost any peripheral nerve, nerve plexus, or spinal nerve can be blocked. Local anesthetic (Lidocaine) block can be done, or this type of block can be modified to include catheter placement for continuous fusion. Permanent blockade may be preferred, eliminating the complications of an indwelling catheter. This can be accomplished with chemical destructive techniques (injecting ethyl alcohol or phenol), radiofrequency lesioning (cutting the nerve), cryoanalgesia (freezing the nerve), botulinum injection, and other techniques. Professional expertise in placing the block is crucial to successful results.

A few common blocks, and the rationale for them, include the following:

- **Trigger point injections**: Well-localized superficial pain
- **Stellate ganglion block**: Upper extremity pain (Pancoast tumor, Raynaud's disease, etc.)
- **Celiac plexus block**: Visceral pain (pancreatic cancer, abdominal metastasis)
- **Lumbar sympathetic block**: Intractable lower extremity pain (neuropathy, leg ulcerations, vascular insufficiency, etc.)
- **Superior hypogastric plexus block**: Pelvic pain (gynecological, colorectal, or genitourinary cancers)
- **Ganglion impar block**: Intractable rectal or perineal pain.

PRECAUTIONS

Blocks are **not a panacea** and have significant **side effects** (3). They should be reserved for those patients in whom pain cannot be controlled adequately by proper administration of systemic analgesics. Blocks do not usually obviate the need for continued systemic analgesics of some kind.

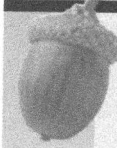

Blocks
IN A NUTSHELL

Nerve blocks are an **option** for patients whose **pain is not controlled** with the WHO ladder of analgesic administration.

Most **all nerves** can be blocked.

Success of the block is directly related to the **expertise** of the professional doing the block; **consultation** is needed.

Systemic analgesics are usually still **needed after** a successful block, but doses are frequently reduced.

Patients should be carefully **assessed** prior to the recommendation of a nerve block.

REFERENCES

1. Swarm RA, Karanikolas M, Cousins MJ. Anaesthetic techniques for pain control. In: Doyle D, Hanks G, Cherny NI, et al., eds. *Oxford Textbook of Palliative Medicine*. 3rd ed. New York: Oxford University Press; 2004:316–341.
2. Mercadante S, Portenoy RK. Opioid poorly-responsive cancer pain. Part I: Clinical considerations. J Pain Symptom Manage. 2001;21:144–150.
3. Reisfield GM, Wilson GR. Blocks of the sympathetic axis for visceral pain. *Fast Facts and Concepts #97*. Milwaukee: The Medical College of Wisconsin; 2002. Available at: http://www.eperc.mcw.edu/fastFact/ff_97.htm. Accessed May 6, 2006.

CHAPTER 80

Addiction vs. Pain

True **addiction is a rare** outcome for patients treated for legitimate pain in end-of-life care (1–3). In the true addict, the level of function is impaired by substance use. However, in the pain patient, the patient's level of function is generally improved with the use of their medication (4).

The **key to preventing barriers** to optimal pain relief is for practitioners to recognize the **difference between** drug **addiction, tolerance**, and **dependency** (5).

TOLERANCE

Definition of tolerance: The need to increase the drug over time to get the same therapeutic effect.

- Significant opioid **tolerance is rare** in pain patients (6).
- Once the correct dose of opioid is obtained, it may stay the same for a long period of time.
- **Increasing dosage** requirements are most likely associated with **progressive disease**.
- **Tolerance** by itself is **not diagnostic** of **addiction**.
- Many drugs (e.g., alcohol, laxatives) produce tolerance.

PHYSICAL DEPENDENCE

Definition of physical dependence: Development of **withdrawal reaction** upon discontinuation or antagonism of the drug.

- **Common** with many drugs (e.g., benzodiazepines, beta-blockers, clonidine, corticosteroids, insulin)!
- Dependence may or may not be present in the pain patient.

- The patient's function is not decreased but may be improved.
- **Dependence** is **not** the same as **addiction**.

PSYCHOLOGICAL ADDICTION

Definition of psychological addition: Overwhelming maladaptive behavior in the acquisition and use of drugs for nonmedical purposes (diversion).

- Continued use in spite of **harm**.
- Patient's **function** is **impaired** rather than enhanced.
- **Loss of control**.
- **Compulsive** drug use.
- Tolerance and physical dependency are common.
- Data suggest that **opioids used to treat pain seldom result in psychological addiction**.

The old idea that "the patient is dying—so what if they get addicted" is neither correct nor very respectful to the patient!

DRUG-SEEKING BEHAVIOR

Unfortunately, clinicians who are legitimately trying to treat pain often fall prey to the manipulations of the drug-seeking patient. Fear of being duped often leads to **under-treating or not treating pain optimally**. A careful **assessment** will help separate the patients who will take their medications responsibly and those who will not. Certainly with time, the pattern of abuse and addiction becomes clear.

Common **risk factors and ploys** of drug-seeking patients include the following, but note that one or two characteristics here do not prove abuse—remember "pseudo-addiction"—but a pattern of behavior is important:

- **History** of substance abuse in the past.
- May **insist** on receiving a controlled medication (of high street value) on the first visit, either stating they are "allergic" to nonaddictive medications or that they "don't work."
- "**Doctor shopping**" and using different pharmacies.
- "Can't afford" or **won't do laboratory or radiological testing** to confirm their pathology.
- Unable to produce old **medical record**; they have varied excuses as to why these cannot be located.
- May claim to have **symptoms** that markedly **deviate from the objective evidence** (history and physical).
- Reports medications are frequently **lost or stolen**—often have very creative explanations of why their medications are missing.

- Other **adverse life consequences**—legal problems and social and family problems.
- Has contact with other people in a **drug culture**—family or friends.
- **Not reliable** in keeping appointments or referrals.
- Does not take the medications as prescribed—frequently takes **extra doses**.
- **Dose escalation** is out of proportion to objective findings.
- Will often **push** the clinician to prescribe when the initial answer is "no." Most physicians do not like confrontation, and good manipulators use that. This is almost always an indication of a scam!
- **Forged or stolen prescriptions**.

SAFEGUARDS

Clinicians should not let the **fear** of being duped or the fear of disciplinary action from regulatory agencies become **barriers** in adequately treating pain (7). There are a number of professional safeguards that minimize these risks:

- Maintain current **knowledge** about treatment of pain and addiction.
- Use a **systematic treatment plan** when using controlled drugs.
- **Document** the **date** when patients receive prescriptions and the **exact amount**.
- Make the **prescriptions hard to alter**—write out the number "Ten" instead of "10," which is easily changed to "100."
- Keep prescription pads and DEA numbers **secure**.
- A written "pain contract" can be helpful in outpatients and other specific cases, but it is usually not necessary with most palliative care patients because they are generally compliant.
- **Document** the patient's **function**.

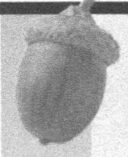

Pain or Addiction?
IN A NUTSHELL

Tolerance: The need to increase the drug to get the same effect.

Physical dependence: Withdrawal occurs if the drug is suddenly stopped.

The presence of opioid tolerance and physical dependence does not equate with "addiction"!

Psychological addiction: Continued use in spite of harm.

Addiction is unusual in pain treatment.

Proper pain treatment makes the patient's function and quality of life better, whereas addiction causes impairment.

REFERENCES

1. Portenoy RK. Opioid therapy for chronic nonmalignant pain: a review of the critical issues, I: special section on opioids for nonmalignant pain. J Pain Symptom Manage. 1996;11:203–217.

2. Savage SR. Opioid use in the management of chronic pain. Med Clin North Am. 1999;83:761–786.

3. Portenoy RK, Payne R. Acute and chronic pain. In: Lowinson JH, Ruiz P, Millman RB, eds. *Substance Abuse: A Comprehensive Textbook.* 2nd ed. Baltimore: Williams & Wilkins; 1992:691–721.

4. Sees KL, Clark HW. Opioid use in the treatment of chronic pain: assessment of addiction. J Pain Symptom Manage. 1993;8:257–264.

5. *AHCPR Archived Clinical Practice Guidelines. Management of cancer pain.* Pharmacologic Management. Available at: http://www.ncbi.nlm.nih.gov/entrez/query.fcgi?cmd=Search&db=books&doptcmdl=GenBookHL&term=addiction,+tolerance+AND+hstat%5Bbook%5D+AND+340638%5Buid%5D&rid=hstat6.section.19028#19047. Accessed May 29, 2006.

6. Foley KM. Changing concepts of tolerance to opioids. In: Chapman CR, Foley KM, eds. *Current and Emerging Issues in Cancer Pain: Research and Practice.* New York: Raven Press; 1993:331–350.

7. Longo LP, Parran T, Johnson B, et al. Addiction: part II. Identification and management of the drug seeking patient. Am Fam Physician. 2000;61:2401–2408.

CHAPTER 81

Pseudo-Addiction

Pseudo-addiction was first described in 1989 to describe a group of patients who took on so-called drug-seeking behaviors as a result of having their **pain undertreated** (1). **Once their pain is adequately treated**, these **behaviors stop** and the **opioids are used responsibly**. Pseudo-addiction is therefore something the **medical profession creates** because of our fear or misunderstanding about pain treatment. True psychological **addiction is extremely low** in medical populations that are taking opioids for legitimate pain (2).

DIAGNOSTIC FEATURES

Uncontrolled pain is a tremendous motivator, and it is easy to understand why patients would go to great lengths to obtain relief. This includes many of the hallmark signs of drug-seeking behavior:

- Seeing more than one clinician to get pain medications refilled.
- Using several pharmacies to fill their scripts.
- Stockpiling or hoarding pain medications for fear of running out.
- Being overly dramatic (moaning, etc.) to demonstrate they are in pain.
- Pain complaints that seem excessive (e.g., answering "14" on the 1 to 10 pain scale!).
- Asking for early refills.
- Clock watching and requesting medication before it is due.
- Stating that their current medication is "like candy" and does not help their pain.

SEPARATING ADDICTION FROM PSEUDO-ADDICTION

If there is suspicion that the patient is addicted or is drug seeking, pseudo-addiction should be **ruled out**. It is important to **assess** the pain (see Chapter 66 on pain assessment) and to review the recent analgesic history. Important points include the following:

- Is this the type of pain that **usually responds** to opioids (somatic or visceral rather than neurogenic)?

- Is the patient getting an **appropriate level** (WHO step 2 or 3) and **dose** of medication?
- Is the **scheduling appropriate**? Are short-acting opioids being ordered every 6, 8, or 12 hours when pharmacology tells us they last only 4 hours?
- Is there a medical or social **history** that suggests previous **substance abuse**?
- **Pseudo-addiction gets better** when appropriate analgesia is prescribed, whereas addiction gets worse.

MANAGEMENT OF PSEUDO-ADDICTION

There are two basic ways to manage pseudo-addiction (3):

- Establish **trust** between the patient and the medical providers. Meet with the patient and **openly discuss** the concerns and **involve the patient** in the decision process about future use of opioids.
- Agree to **prescribe opioids** at pharmacologically **appropriate doses** and **time intervals**. Escalate the dose until analgesia is maintained or side effects develop (see Chapter 68 on dose escalation). Reevaluate the patient: If the drug-seeking behavior does not subside, suspect true addiction.

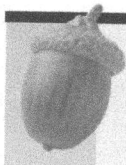

Pseudo-Addiction
IN A NUTSHELL

Pseudo-addiction is a term that applies to the drug-seeking behaviors of patients whose **pain is being undertreated**.

These **behaviors go away** when the pain is **adequately treated**.

Pseudo-addiction should be **ruled out** in any patient suspected of being addicted or drug seeking.

True **addiction is rare** in legitimate pain patients.

Pseudo-addiction is **managed** by **openly discussing** the situation with the patient or by **providing appropriate analgesia** for the patient.

REFERENCES

1. Weissman DE, Haddox JD. Opioid pseudoaddiction: an iatrogenic syndrome. Pain. 1989;36:363–366.
2. Aronoff GM. Letters—medical treatment of opiate addiction. JAMA. 2000;283:2931.
3. Weissman DE. Pseudoaddiction. *Fast Facts and Concepts #69*. Milwaukee: Medical College of Wisconsin; 2002. Available at: http://www.eperc.mcw.edu/fastFact/ff_69.htm. Accessed April 22, 2006.

Palliative Interventions

CHAPTER 82

Tube Feeding in Palliative Care

In our culture, **feeding and nutrition** are often linked to **nurturing**, love, and affection. Therefore great concern arises when a patient cannot or will not eat. Tube feeding is frequently seen as an alternative. However, the evidence shows feeding tubes to be ineffective, except in a few specific situations. As always, in palliative care, the **patient's goals must be considered**.

Goal: To prolong life in acute situations

Data for tube feeding are **strongest** for patients with reversible illness (1).

- Proximal GI obstruction and a high functional status
- Patients receiving chemotherapy involving proximal GI tract
- Certain patients with AIDS and wasting syndromes

Goal: To prolong life in chronic disease

Data are **weakest** in advanced cancer, dementia, and patients with multiple co-morbidities:

- Anorexia and dysphagia are often markers of **severe multisystem disease** and carry a high mortality rate in spite of artificial feeding (2).
- **No survival advantage** of tube feeding has been found in patients with **advanced dementia** (3).
- Nutrition from feeding tubes **does not** prevent or increase the healing **of pressure ulcers, improve function**, or **extend life** in chronic illness.

Goal: To prevent aspiration

- **No study** has shown a **reduction of aspiration pneumonia** with tube feeding (4).
- Numerous **observational studies** demonstrate a **higher incidence** of **aspiration pneumonia** in those who have been tube fed.

Goal: To improve comfort

- **No studies** have demonstrated **improved quality of life**.
- Feeding tubes may **adversely affect quality of life** through increased need for physical restraints, infections, pain, indignity, cost, and the denial of the pleasure of eating (5).

Swallowing Studies

- Evidence indicates that swallowing studies may be helpful in providing swallowing instructions and techniques to cognitive patients.
- In **impaired patients, swallowing studies** such as videofluoroscopy **lack both sensitivity and specificity** in predicting who will develop aspiration pneumonia (6).

Alternatives to Feeding Tubes

- **Hand feeding** allows the maintenance of patient comfort and intimate patient care during the natural decline in end of life.
- Use **strategies to improve food intake**: strong flavors of foods; alter the amounts, consistency, and availability of food.
- **Educate the family** and staff that not eating is a normal facet of the dying process and not the cause. **No evidence** indicates that **not eating** is **distressful to the patient or causes any suffering**.

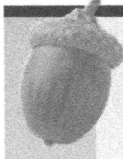

Tube Feeding in Palliative Care
IN A NUTSHELL

All dying patients eventually develop an **unwillingness to eat and drink**.

Tube feeding should be considered only after exploring the **patient's goals**.

No evidence indicates that tube feedings in patients at the end of life prolong life, add comfort, prevent aspiration pneumonia, or improve functional status.

Some **disadvantages** of feeding tubes include the loss of pleasure from eating, cost, and the need for increased physical and chemical restraints, increased infections, increased aspiration, and loss of dignity.

Swallowing studies lack both sensitivity and specificity.

REFERENCES

1. Withholding and withdrawing life-sustaining treatment. Am Fam Physician. 2000. Updated July 2005. Available at: http://www.aafp.org/afp/20001001/1555.html. Accessed June 11, 2006.
2. Cowen ME, Simpson S, Vettere T. Survival estimates for patients with abnormal swallowing studies. J Gen Intern Med. 1997;12:88–94.

3. Ina LI. Feeding tubes in patients with severe dementia. Am Fam Physician. 2002;65: 1605–1610.
4. Finucane TE, Bynum JP. Use of tube feeding to prevent aspiration pneumonia. Lancet. 1996;348:1421–1424.
5. Ahronheim JC. Nutrition and hydration in the terminal patient. Clin Geriatr. 1996;12: 379–391.
6. Croghan JE, Burke EM, Caplan S, et al. Pilot study of 12-month outcomes of nursing home patients with aspiration on videofluoroscopy. Dysphagia. 1994;9:141–146.

CHAPTER 83

Palliative Chemotherapy

Palliative chemotherapy is antitumor therapy used **solely for symptom control and not for cure** (1). Several agents are now available that may meet this goal in certain selected cancers and hosts (2). As always in palliative care, the **patient's goals** are the deciding factor.

PATIENT SELECTION

Patients interested in palliative chemotherapy may have unreasonable expectations and overestimate the benefits of the treatment. Therefore it is important to **assess the patient well**. Here are important factors to consider:

- What is the patient's **goal**?
- Explore the patient's **emotional, spiritual**, and **social domains**.
- If the request to pursue palliative chemotherapy is based on **anecdotal experiences** or the patient just "**wanting to try something**," it is to be **discouraged**.
- **Communication** with the patient should be centered around:
    - the likelihood of **response**.
    - treatment-related **toxicities**.
    - the expected impact on **quality of life**.
    - **the length of time** chemotherapy will be needed.
- Make clear to the patient and family that this is **not intended to be curative** because many patients may hold on to this hope.

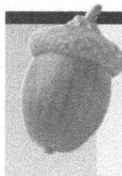

Palliative Chemotherapy
IN A NUTSHELL

Palliative chemotherapy is for **symptom control and not for cure.** It may be appropriate for certain conditions and patients.

The patient's **goals** must be considered.

A favorable response depends on careful **patient selection** and on **close collaboration between the oncologist and the palliative care specialist.**

REFERENCES

1. Ellison NM, Chevlin EM. Palliative chemotherapy. In: Berger AM, Portenoy RK, Weissman DE, eds. *Principles and Practice of Supportive Oncology.* 2nd ed. Philadelphia: Lippincott Williams & Wilkins; 2002.
2. Prommer E. Guidelines for the use of palliative chemotherapy. Am Acad Hospice Palliat Med Bull. 2004;5:1–13.

CHAPTER 84

Palliative Radiation

Radiation can be used in malignancies with a goal to improve **quality of life** by **reducing pain, increasing function**, or **relieving pressure on a vital structure**. Between 25% and 40% of radiation is now used for symptom control in otherwise incurable cancer—palliation rather than cure (1).

INDICATIONS

Common **cancer syndromes** in which radiation therapy is palliative include the following (2):

- Painful **bone metastasis**
- **Spinal cord compression**
- **Superior vena cava syndrome**—dyspnea, orthopnea, and venous congestion secondary to tumor impingement
- **Brain metastasis**
- **Obstruction** of the esophagus, airway, biliary tract, and so on

PATIENT SELECTION

As with any palliative therapy, the patient should be **well assessed**. It should be emphasized that this is **not curative**, to prevent false hope. Here are other important factors to consider (3):

- What is the patient's **goal** for therapy?
- What is the expected **response rate**? Is it likely to improve function or quality of life?
- What are the expected **toxicities** and **side effects**?
- What is the **treatment burden** (e.g., cost, time spent coming to and from therapy, number of treatments, time off work for family, etc.)?

SPECIFIC TREATMENTS

In general, radiation therapy can be **very effective** in relieving appropriate symptoms. Common treatments include the following (4):

- **External beam radiation**—from outside the body. After mapping a target, most palliative patients receive radiation doses for a very short time each day, 5 days per week for 1 to 3 weeks. Toxicity depends on the area being treated.
- **Radionuclide injection**—Strontium 89 or Samarium 153 are indicated for multiple-site bone metastases. Peak effect is at 3 to 6 weeks (so a prognosis of at least that long is essential). A worsening pain flare may occur prior to relief. Toxicity is usually hematologic with decreased blood counts.
- **Combination** of preceding therapies.

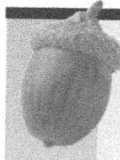

Palliative Radiation
IN A NUTSHELL

Palliative radiation is for symptom control and **not for cure.** Results may be good for appropriate patients.

Indications include painful bone metastases, brain metastases, or tumor pressure on any vital structure.

The **patient's goals**, prognosis, expected results, and treatment burden must be carefully considered.

External beam radiation and **radionuclide** injection are common methods of receiving radiation.

REFERENCES

1. Lutz S, Conner S. Radiation oncology and hospice: cornerstones in palliative care. Am Acad Hospice Palliat Med Bull. Spring 2005;6:1–3.
2. Tisdale BA. When to consider radiation therapy for your patient. Am Fam Physician. 1999;59;1177–1189.
3. Rutter C, Weissman DE. Radiation for palliation—Part 2. *Fast Facts and Concepts #67.* End-of-Life Physician Education Resource Center; 2002. Available at: www.eperc.mcw.edu. Accessed June 25, 2006.
4. Kirkbride P. The role of radiation therapy in palliative care. J Palliat Care. 1995;11:19–26.

CHAPTER 85

"Response Rate" in Cancer Chemotherapy

It is helpful for the patient and the clinician to fully understand *response rate* when talking to palliative care patients about chemotherapy and goal setting.

RESPONSE RATE OF CHEMOTHERAPY

This is the oncologic definition of *response rate* (1): Complete responders + partial responders/total number of patients treated.

$$\frac{\text{Complete Responders} + \text{Partial Responders}}{\text{Total Number of Patients Treated}} = \text{Response Rate}$$

Definitions

- Complete responders: complete eradication of measurable tumor.

- Partial responders: reduction in tumor size of at least 50% lasting 1 month or more.

- Response is usually determined after two cycles of treatment.

- If a clinical trial shows "0" complete responders (eradication of tumor), but half of the patients experienced a 50% or greater reduction in tumor size for 1 month, before it begins to grow again, the response rate quoted to the patient is 50%. Patients and clinicians alike may interpret that as meaning a 50% cure rate, which may be far from true.

- Response rate data come from clinical trials using good performance status and highly monitored patients. In general, the response rates for patients outside of the trials can be expected to be lower.

MEDIAN DURATION OF RESPONSE

The *median duration of response* is also important for the patient to understand to make an informed decision about chemotherapy. This number is how long the response lasts:

- Duration of response may be as short as 1 to 2 months for chemotherapy in pancreatic cancer, to 9 to 12 months in some breast cancer treatments.

MEDIAN SURVIVAL

- The *median survival* includes both responders and nonresponders and is an important figure for patients contemplating initiating or continuing chemotherapy.

For examples of response rates, see Table 15.

TABLE 15

Typical Response Rates, Median Duration of Response, and Median Survival Numbers for Typical Cancers Treated with Chemotherapy

Cancer Type	Response Rate	Median Duration of Response	Median Survival
Breast	25%–55%	6–12 mo	24–36 mo
Colon	25%–35%	6–8 mo	12–18 mo
Lung: Non–Small Cell	20%–30%	4–6 mo	6–9 mo
Esophagus	30%–50%	4–6 mo	6–9 mo
Stomach	20%–30%	4–6 mo	6–9 mo
Melanoma	15%–25%	4–6 mo	6–9 mo
Pancreas	15%–25%	3–5 mo	6–9 mo
Liver (Hepatoma)	5%–15%	2–4 mo	6–9 mo
Biliary	5%–15%	2–4 mo	6–9 mo

From Weissman DE, von Gunten CF. Chemotherapy: response and survival data. *Fast Facts and Concepts #99.* End-of-Life Physicians Education Resource Center; October 2003. Available at: http://www.eperc.mcw.edu/fastFact/ff_099.htm. Accessed June 12, 2006.

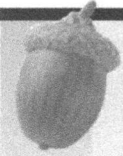

"Response Rate" in Cancer Chemotherapy
IN A NUTSHELL

Response rate, duration of response, and median survival are all important factors to understand when talking to patients about prognosis and goal setting regarding chemotherapy.

REFERENCE

1. Ellison NM, Chevlin EM. Palliative chemotherapy. In: Berger AM, Portenoy RK, Weissman DE, eds. *Principles and Practice of Supportive Oncology.* 2nd ed. Philadelphia: Lippincott Williams & Wilkins; 2002.

CHAPTER 86

Ventilator Withdrawal

Ethically and legally there is **no difference** between **withholding and withdrawing** mechanical ventilator support for a patient who has reached end of life (1). Actually, the moral weight may favor withdrawing life support because of the added knowledge of a poor prognosis after a therapeutic trial on the ventilator has been completed (2).

PREPARING THE FAMILY AND STAFF

At the end-of-life, the **goal** in **withdrawing** mechanical ventilator support is to **allow a natural death**. The **patient is the authority** in these decisions (3). This is a very difficult and emotionally charged resolution for the family, so **proper preparation is essential**:

- **Never assume** what the family and medical staff understand. Discuss removing life support in a **simple and clear manner** (see Chapter 13 on family meetings). Make it **very clear** that the patient will most likely **die** when life support is stopped. **Communication is key**! Don't forget to talk to the staff because they often have a bond with their patient and need to understand why this is occurring.

- Explain to those present that **involuntary movement or gasping may occur** but that it is natural and **not a sign of suffering**. Assure them the patient will be kept comfortable.

- Plan for **family members, clergy, staff, or anyone else** that the family requests to be at the bedside.

- Assure the family that they may **provide music, religious symbols, or rituals** that are important to them—be **respectful** of their wishes and **culture**.

- Make sure amenities such as **tissues** and adequate seating is available for the family or staff.

- **Document** clinical findings and discussions.

PREPARING THE PATIENT

Once the decision has been confirmed, and everyone is ready, begin preparing the patient. Your **goal is for a peaceful death**. A number of simple actions will make the experience less devastating and assure that things go smoothly:

- **Turn off all monitors and alarms**: Alarms going off are very upsetting to the family.
- **Remove unnecessary apparatus** from the patient such as oxygen monitors, and so on (**IV access will be needed**). It is usually better to leave arterial lines, NG tubes, catheters, and so on, in place until after the patient is pronounced dead. Their removal may be perceived as painful or contributing to the patient's death.

PREPARING YOURSELF

This is one of the **most difficult things we do** in medicine. Yet, if done properly, it is an **opportunity to lessen the trauma to all those involved**:

- **Be firm** in your decision: Loved ones are often looking for the smallest clue that this is not happening. Any perceived hesitancy on the part of the clinician may give false hope or create anxiety.
- **Be prepared**: Rehearse the extubation in your mind and have all the necessary medication available at the bedside. Sending to the pharmacy for more IV morphine while the family is watching their loved one moan and gasp for air is devastating and destroys your professionalism.
- **Leadership of the clinician is crucial**: You may need to keep reassuring the family that this is "the right thing."
- It is **okay to be somber** and to even **show appropriate emotion**. You are human; this is hard to do; and the family will respect that.
- **Get help**: Having an experienced physician at the bedside is reassuring to everyone. It is also helpful to have a respiratory therapist at the bedside and a skilled nurse to assist.

REMOVING THE VENTILATOR

There are two standard methods for removing the ventilator. The clinician's judgment, the patient's comfort, and the family's perception will determine which method is best for each individual person:

Immediate extubation: After appropriate suctioning the endotracheal tube (ET) is removed and the patient is placed on humidified oxygen by mask.

Terminal weaning: The ventilator rate, pressure, and oxygen levels are slowly decreased with the ET left in place. This may be done over 30 to 60 minutes or several hours. The following protocol (for adult patients) (4–6) can be used with either method.

PROTOCOL

Sedation should be provided to **all patients**, even those that are comatose:

- Consider placing **two scopolamine patches** or giving **glycopyrrolate, 0.4 to 0.8 mg IV** (adult dosing), 30 to 60 minutes prior to extubation to decrease secretions.
- **Discontinue** any **paralytics** that may be running.
- Administer a **2- to 10-mg bolus of morphine IV** push.
- Begin a **continuous morphine infusion at 50%** of the bolus dose per hour.
- Give **midazolam (Versed), 1 to 2 mg IV**.
- Start a **midazolam (Versed) continuous infusion at 1 mg per hour**.
- In the conscious patient, **titrate** the just cited infusion rates of MS and Versed as needed to control anxiety and achieve **maximum comfort prior to extubation**.
- **Have additional IV medication** drawn up **at the bedside** to give if needed for symptom relief.
- Set the F_{IO_2} to 21%. Watch for respiratory distress and **adjust the medication** if needed to make the patient comfortable before continuing.
- If the patient is comfortable, **suction well**—both the ET tube and oral secretions.
- Have a nurse or **assistant on the opposite side of the bed** with a **towel or wash-cloth and an oral suction catheter**.
- **Deflate the cuff** on the ET tube.
- **Remove the ET** under the clean towel, and wrap the tube to keep it and the usual secretions covered.
- Have someone assigned to take the tube, towel, and all the hoses, along with the **ventilator, out of the room**. Remember to turn off the ventilator and all alarms.
- **Suction** again if necessary.
- **Encourage the family to hold the patient's hand, touch**, and **provide assurances** to their loved one.
- If the patient has breathing efforts, **oxygen may be placed by mask**, according to the family's wishes.
- **Spend some time**: Many patients will have spontaneous respirations for a while until they tire. Be prepared and **assure the family this is normal** and the patient is **not suffering**.
- After death, **encourage the family to spend as much time** as required at the bedside.
- Provide **grief support** and **follow-up bereavement support**.
- **Gather your staff** away from the family and **discuss (debrief)** how the removal of life support went. Let everyone express their feelings.

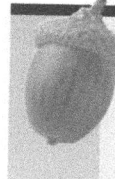

Ventilator Withdrawal
IN A NUTSHELL

The **patient is the authority** in making the decision to remove ventilator support. If the patient is not decisional, the question to the family is "What would the patient want?"

Preparation is essential: Prepare the family; prepare the patient; and prepare yourself!

Decide on a method of removing the ventilator: **immediate extubation** or **terminal weaning**.

All patients should receive sedation, even if the patient is comatose!

Follow something similar to the **medical protocol** presented in this chapter.

Communicate and plan for **follow-up**.

REFERENCES

1. Heffner JE. Chronic obstructive pulmonary disease. Respir Care Clin N Am. 1998; 4:345–358.
2. Heffner JE. End-of-life ethical issues. Respir Care Clin N Am. 1998;4:541–559.
3. Henig NR, Faul JL, Raffin TA. Biomedical ethics and the withdrawal of advanced life support. Annu Rev Med. 2001;52:79–92.
4. Emanuel LL, von Gunten CF, Ferris FF, eds. Module 11: withholding and withdrawing therapy. In: *The EPEC Curriculum: Education for Physicians on End-of-Life Care.* The EPEC Project; 1999.
5. Rubenfeld GD, Crawford SW. Principles and practice of withdrawing life-sustaining treatment in the ICU. In: Curtis JR, Rubenfeld GD, eds. *Managing Death in the Intensive Care Unit.* New York: Oxford University Press; 2001:127–147.
6. Rubenfeld GD. Principles and practice of withdrawing life-sustaining treatments. Crit Care Clin. 2004;3:435–451.

CHAPTER 87

Bowel Obstruction

Malignant bowel obstruction occurs frequently in conditions such as ovarian and colon cancers. **Symptoms** are usually **obvious** from physical examination and are easily confirmed on a plain abdominal radiograph (air-fluid levels seen) if the diagnosis is in doubt.

SURGICAL MANAGEMENT

Surgical palliation is a very **complex decision** and must be carefully measured on each individual patient. Depending on the patient's overall **medical condition, prognosis, quality of life, and goals**, surgical options can be considered:

- **Surgical correction**: removal of the obstruction and reanastomosis of the intestine. This is major surgery and should be reserved for patients who have a good life expectancy and have had a good preobstruction quality of life (1).
- Placement of a **diverting ostomy** (stoma).
- Placement of a **stent** across the obstructed site.
- Placing a **venting tube**, such as a gastrostomy tube, colon tube, NG tube, and so on.

> **The dying patient should be spared from the traditional IV fluids and NG tube ("drip and suck").**

MEDICAL MANAGEMENT

Medications are now available that focus on the relief of symptoms in malignant bowel obstruction:

- Colicky pain secondary to smooth muscle spasm and bowel wall distension:
  - **Octreotide (Sandostatin**): Gives symptomatic relief by inhibiting peristalsis. Octreotide has rapidly become the **drug of choice** in malignant bowel

obstruction because of limited side effects. Administered as a SC injection (starting at 50 to 100 μg every 8 hours) or as a continuous IV or SC infusion (beginning at 10 to 20 μg per hour). The medication is titrated every 24 hours until abdominal pain, nausea, and vomiting are controlled (2). Most palliative care patients respond to 200 μg every 8 hours or less (3).

- **Opioids**: Titrate to pain. Some studies indicate that **fentanyl** and **methadone** may be better tolerated than morphine in GI obstruction because morphine tends to accumulate in intestinal tissue (4,5).

- **Antisecretory** medications: Scopolamine (parenteral at 10 μg per hour SC/IV continuous infusion or transdermal patch (10 μg per hour); glycopyrrolate (0.1 to 0.2 mg SC or IV three or four times per day).

- **Corticosteroids**: May reduce bowel obstruction secondary to decreasing inflammatory changes in the bowel wall (6).

- Nausea and vomiting (see Chapter 49)

  - Metoclopramide (Reglan): May be helpful in partial obstruction but may exacerbate symptoms in complete obstruction (dose: 10 mg SC every 4 hours).

  - Prochlorperazine (Compazine): 5 to 10 mg SC or IV every 4 hours.

  - Promethazine (Phenergan): 12.5 to 50 mg IV or SC every 4 to 6 hours.

  - Haloperidol (Haldol): 0.5 to 5.0 mg SC or IV every 8 to 12 hours (avoid IV administration)

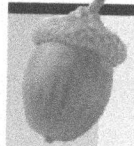

Bowel Obstruction
IN A NUTSHELL

Surgical therapy is limited in palliative care patients and should be carefully evaluated according to the patient's goals of care. It should be considered only for those with a good quality of life and excellent prognosis.

Octreotide (Sandostatin) has become the **first-line drug** for supportive medical management of bowel obstruction in the palliative care patient.

Other **symptoms** can be controlled with opioids, antisecretory medications, corticosteroids, and medication for nausea and vomiting.

REFERENCES

1. Sainsbury R, Vaizey C, Pastorino U, et al. Surgical palliation. In: Doyle D, Hanks G, Cherny N, et al., eds. *Oxford Textbook of Palliative Medicine*. 3rd ed. New York: Oxford University Press; 2004:255–266.
2. Mercadante S, Ferrera P, Villari P, et al. Aggressive pharmacological treatment for reversing malignant bowel obstruction. J Pain Symptom Manage. 2004;28:412–416.
3. Taylor GJ, Kurent JE. *A Clinician's Guide to Palliative Care*. 2003. Malden, Mass: Blackwell; 2003:44.

4. Mercadante S. What is the opioid of choice? Prog Palliat Care. 2001;9:190–193.
5. Mercadante S, Sapio M, Serretta R. Treatment of pain in chronic bowel obstruction with self-administration or methadone. Support Care Cancer. 1997;5:327–329.
6. Feuer DJ, Broadley KE. Corticosteroids for the resolution of malignant bowel obstruction in advanced gynaecological and gastrointestinal cancer. Cochrane Database Syst Rev. 2000; (2):CD001219. Review.

CHAPTER 88

Treating the Death Rattle

Few things are as disturbing to the caregivers and family during the actively dying phase as the so-called **death rattle**, caused by the dying person's inability to swallow normal oral secretions, **pooling of the secretions**, and resultant gurgling with respirations. However, **no evidence** indicates this is **uncomfortable** for the patient (1) any more than **snoring** is to the person doing the snoring.

NONPHARMACOLOGICAL TREATMENTS

A few simple actions may help:

- Change the patient's **position** by laying the patient on his or her side or in a semi-prone position to encourage postural drainage. Even a brief trial of Trendelenburg might help.
- Gentle oropharyngeal **suctioning** may help, but secretions may be beyond the reach of the catheter. Vigorous and frequent suctioning is probably more distressing than the rattle.

PHARMACOLOGICAL TREATMENTS

The onset of the death rattle is a **good predictor** of very limited life expectancy, usually less than 16 hours (2). Therefore concern about significant side effects from medications is limited when compared to the goal of care.

Common effective **medications include** the following:

- **Atropine eye drops** 1%, 1 to 2 drops sublingually, titrated every 30 minutes as needed.
- **Scopolamine patches**, one or two applied every 3 days (onset is slower than other forms of administration). Write "for palliative care" on the prescription if two patches are given at once, or the pharmacy may not fill it.
- **Levsin solution (hyoscyamine)**, 0.125 mg per mL. 1 mL (0.125 mg) PO titrated every 30 minutes as needed (3).

- **Glycopyrrolate (Robinul)**, 0.2 to 0.8 mg SC or IV every 4 to 8 hours to titrate. (Notice the wide range of titration. Glycopyrrolate given IV with be effective in 1 to 2 minutes, so giving small amounts every few minutes and titrating to response is an effective method. Glycopyrrolate is five times stronger than atropine in drying secretions.)

COMMUNICATION

Communicating with the family may be more important at this point than treating the patient. Explain that the patient is actively dying. **Symptoms often escalate as death approaches**, and even families that are well informed may begin to question their ability to handle the situation (4). Families often have an interpretation of the death rattle that may or may not be distressful (5). See Chapter 38, "The Syndrome of Imminent Death."

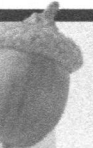

Death Rattle
IN A NUTSHELL

The **death rattle** is caused by breathing pooled secretions and is predictive of actively dying.

The death rattle is probably **not uncomfortable** to the patient, but it is often treated for the sake of the family and caregivers.

Positional changes may be helpful.

Medications include:

    Atropine eye drops 0.1%, 1 to 2 drops sublingually every 30 minutes as needed

    Scopolamine transdermal patches, one or two every 3 days

    Levsin (hyoscyamine), 0.125 mg every 30 minutes as needed

    Glycopyrrolate, 0.2 to 0.8 mg IV or SC every 4 to 8 hours as needed

REFERENCES

1. Bickel K, Arnold R. Death rattle and oral secretions. *Fast Facts and Concepts #109*. End-of-Life Physician Education Resource Center; March 2004. Available at: www.eperc.mcw.edu.
2. Wilders H, Menten J. Death rattle: prevalence, prevention and treatment. J Pain Symptom Manage. 2002;23:310–317.
3. *Epocrates ID*. Version 2.70. Updated May 30, 2006.
4. Taylor GJ, Kurent JE. *A Clinician's Guide to Palliative Care*. Malden, Mass: Blackwell; 2003.
5. Wee Bl, Coleman PG, Hillier R, et al. The sound of death rattle II: how do relatives interpret the sound? Palliat Med. 2006;20:177–181.

CHAPTER 89

Aggressive Wound Treatment

The ultimate goals of treating pressure ulcer/wounds at the end of life is for pain control, to manage infection, odor, bleeding, and exudates, and to maintain patient dignity and quality of life for the patient and caregiver (1). Traditionally, wounds on the terminally ill were treated by applying a dressing and trying to address the pain systemically. However, wounds that are treated **topically** and **aggressively** can respond well. Anecdotal reports over a 4-year period show a resolution rate close to 40%.

STAGING OF WOUND DAMAGE

Stage 1

- Nonblanching erythema of intact skin
- Heralding lesion of skin ulceration
- Darker skin, discoloration; red, blue, or purple hues
- Warmth, edema, induration, or hardness as indicators

Stage 2

- Partial-thickness skin loss involving epidermis, dermis, or both
- Ulcer is superficial
- Presents clinically as an abrasion, blister, or shallow crater

Stage 3

- Full-thickness skin loss involving damage or necrosis of subcutaneous tissue that may extend down to underlying fascia
- Ulcer presents clinically as a deep crater with or without undermining of adjacent tissue

255

Stage 4

- Full-thickness skin loss with extensive destruction, tissue necrosis, or damage to muscle, bone, or supporting structures
- Undermining and sinus tracts also may be associated (2,3,4)

STAGES OF HEALING

Inflammation: 1 to 5 days

- White blood cells help in cleaning wound
- Macrophages signal growth factors

Proliferative Phase: 5 to 25 days

- Granulation: Angiogenesis; red, beefy appearance
- Epithelization: Cells slide into and across wound bed
- Contraction: Wound shrinks; changes size and/or shape

Maturation: 25 days to 2 years

- Scar tissue strengthens
- Lysis of collagen fibers
- Synthesis of new collagen fibers
- Only 80% normal strength regained (1,2,4)

CLEANSING WOUNDS

Wounds should be cleaned using only **federally** approved cleansers including:

- Normal saline or **wound cleanser** with PSI 4 to 16
- Do *not* use iodine, Betadine, peroxide, or topical antiseptics:
  - They are **cytoxic** to fibroblasts and new skin (4)
  - It is considered **fraud** and **outside standards of care** to use these preparations (6)

DRESSINGS

Choose the **appropriate dressings**:

- Dry wound; keep moist.
- Heavy exudates: use absorptive dressing.
- Avoid frequent dressing changes. Changing a dressing once per week can be enough!
- With each dressing change, 4 hours of healing time is lost secondary to **shock** and loss of new tissue.
- **Fill** any **depth** with loose packing.
- Use a cover dressing to protect the wound from further trauma (1,2,5).

INFECTION

Redness, warmth, erythema, and pain are signs and symptoms of inflammation, *not* infection. If infection is suspected:

- Infection can be from fungus, virus, or bacteria.
- Culture the wound: Swabs are not effective and often cultures only necrotic tissue that may contain a number of pathogens. Needle biopsy is more accurate. Punch biopsy is the most accurate.
- Apply topical antibiotic for local infection (4):
  - Metronidazole 20%/Lidocaine 25 with 78% Polyox powder:
  - Kills smell
  - Relieves pain
  - Kills aerobic and anaerobic bacteria
  - Silver products also kill gram-positive and gram-negative bacteria:
- Releases silver over 7-day period

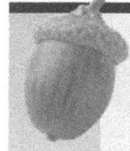

Aggressive Wound Management
IN A NUTSHELL

Pressure ulcers and wounds are common in populations with advanced disease but can be managed or healed.

Staging of the wound provides a standard description of wound severity and provides a reference for wound healing.

Avoid iodine, Betadine, peroxide, and other harsh chemicals that destroy new skin cells.

Apply appropriate dressings.

Redness, warmth, erythema, and pain indicate inflammation not infection.

REFERENCES

1. Bryant R. Acute and chronic wounds. In: *Nursing Management*. 2nd ed. St. Louis: Mosby; 2000.
2. Emory University. *Wound, Ostomy and Continence Nursing Education Program: Skin and Wound Module*. 3rd ed. September 2002.
3. Hess CT. *Clinical Guide to Wound Care*. 4th ed. Springhouse, Pa: Springhouse Corporation.
4. *Quick Reference Guide for Clinicians: #15, Pressure Ulcer Treatment*. U.S. Department of Health and Human Services; December 1994.
5. Afflerbach D. Wound Care Seminar, Manuel: 2002–2003.
6. Hogue E. Legal: five crucial legal issues for homecare providers. Remington Report. 2003; 11:b22.

The Palliative Pediatric Patient

CHAPTER 90

Children and Death

Children who are dying know it (1). They are not dependent on information from parents or health care personnel. Studies agree that by 7 years of age, children can understand the death concepts of universality, irreversibility, no functionality, and causality (2). These concepts can be integrated with the child's developmental age and level (Table 16) (3,4).

TABLE 16

Children's Concepts of Death

Stage of Development	Key Concepts	Example	Practical Implications
Infancy	Experience the world through sensory information Death is perceived as separation or abandonment Protest and despair from disruption in caretaking	Aware of tension, the unfamiliar, and separation	Comfort by sensory input (touch, rocking, sucking) and familiar people as well as transitional objects (toys)
Early verbal childhood (2–6 yr)	See death as reversible or temporary Magical thinking that wishes can come true Death may be seen as punishment	Do not believe death could happen to them May equate death with sleep May believe they can cause death by their thoughts, such as wishing someone would go away	Provide concrete information about state of being (e.g., "A dead person no longer breathes or eats.") Need to dispel concept of being responsible and therefore guilty because of thoughts
Middle childhood (7–12 yr)	Personalize death Aware that death is final Earlier stage: understand causality by external causes	Aware that death can happen to them Believe that death is caused by an event, such as an accident	Child may request graphic details about death, including burial and decomposition

(continued)

TABLE 16 (Continued)

Children's Concepts of Death

Stage of Development	Key Concepts	Example	Practical Implications
	Later stage: understand causality by internal causes	Understand that death also can be caused by an illness	May benefit from specifics about an illness
Adolescence (>12 yr)	Appreciate universality of death but may feel distanced from it	May engage in risky behavior, stating "It can't happen to me" or "Everyone dies anyway"	May have a need to speak about unrealized plans, such as schooling and marriage

Modified from American Academy of Pediatrics, Committee on Psychosocial Aspects of Child and Family Health. The pediatrician and childhood bereavement. Pediatrics. 2000;105:445–447, and Perkin RM, Swift JD, Raper JT. *Primer on Pediatric Palliative Care.* Greenville, NC: University Printing and Graphics of East Carolina University Press; 2005.

END-OF-LIFE COMMUNICATION FOR CHILDREN

One of the most difficult aspects of pediatric palliative care is communication. To ensure the child's preferences about treatments are adequately addressed, documented, and followed, the health care team must use effective communication (5):

- Majority of parents do want information and they want it from their physician
- Difficult conversations are more manageable if they are seen as a process
- Careful planning and consensus development: Remember cultural considerations
- **Preferred setting**:
  - Quiet
  - Comfortable
  - Convenient time
  - Sufficient time
  - Private
  - Support person(s) for parent(s)
  - Other members of health care team
  - Provide tissue
- **Physician obstacles**:
  - Conflict with perceived role of curing, prolonging life, and improving health
  - Lack of education or formal training
  - Stress around the delivery of bad news
  - Sense of failure surrounding treatment efforts
  - Loss of relationship with the patient and the investment in his or her care
- **Specific fears related to the delivery of bad news**:
  - Fear of being blamed
  - Fear of how the child/family will react

- Fear of expressing emotion or breaching "professional" conduct
- Fear of not knowing the answers

- **Value of skilled conversations**:
  - Shift focus of care from cure or prolongation of life to skilled palliative care
  - Improved management of the child's pain and other symptoms
  - Decreased stress

- **Talking with the dying child**:
  - Most children with a life-threatening illness or condition have a greater understanding of what death means than do healthy children their own age
  - Terminally ill children are usually aware of their prognoses, even if they take great pains to hide that knowledge from the adults around them
  - Terminally ill children feel less isolated if they can communicate their concerns
  - Stay open and receptive when the child initiates a conversation
  - Recognize that many children communicate best through nonverbal means, such as artwork or music
  - Reassure continued love and physical closeness and minimization of pain
  - Respect the child's need to be alone

- **Children's understanding of death**:
  - Providing emotional and psychological support for the dying child is as important as providing relief of physical symptoms
  - Parents frequently have many questions about how much the child perceives of the terminal condition and how to be most supportive in allaying the child's fears and any misconceptions
  - Parents are often struggling to meet the emotional needs of siblings
  - Palliative care team can support the parents' efforts by providing education on child's normal developmental understanding of death

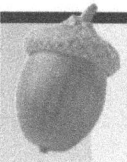

Children and Death
IN A NUTSHELL

Children who are dying know it!

Communication skills with children in palliative care are one of the most difficult but also the most important aspects of care.

Most parents, and children, want honest information.

REFERENCES

1. Martinson ID. Improving care of dying children. West J Med. 1995;163:258–262.
2. Speece MW, Brent SB. The development of children's understanding of death. In: Corr CA, Corr DM, eds. *Handbook of childhood death and bereavement*. New York: Springer; 1996:29–50.

3. Frager G. Children's concepts of death. In: Joishy SK, ed. *Palliative Medicine Secrets.* Philadelphia: Hanley & Belfus; 1999:170–171.
4. American Academy of Pediatrics, Committee on Psychosocial Aspects of Child and Family Health. The pediatrician and childhood bereavement. Pediatrics. 2000;105:445–447.
5. Perkin RM, Swift JD, Raper JT. *Primer on Pediatric Palliative Care.* Greenville, NC: University Printing and Graphics of East Carolina University Press; 2005.

CHAPTER 91

Neonatal Population

When parents lose an infant, they are losing more than a child. They are losing their hopes and dreams for the future. The health care team must help the family focus on the positive aspects of the infant's life, no matter how short. Support from the health care team can include these actions:

- Encourage the family to name the infant and hold the infant, regardless of presence of congenital malformations.
- Support religious rituals such as baptism and pastoral counseling.
- Foster memories by providing photographs (especially in the parent's arms), footprints, and locks of hair.
- Help the family plan for autopsy, organ donation, disposition of the body, and funeral arrangements.
- Work with families to explain the death to the infant's siblings (1). Child life specialists are a valuable resource trained to work with siblings.
- Counsel the family about the cause of death and risk for future pregnancies and help answer the questions (spoken or not spoken).

PAIN CONTROL

The parents of a dying infant experience a variety of emotions ranging from denial to guilt, but their primary fear is that their child will experience pain. It is inhumane to let infants suffer from pain without appropriate intervention (Table 17) (2,3). Unique challenges regarding pain in neonates include the following:

- The difficulty of confidently diagnosing pain in this vulnerable population.
- Objective quantification of infant pain is generally based on recognizing the infant's responses to pain via physiologic changes (i.e., change in heart rate, blood pressure, or oxygen saturation) or behavioral responses (i.e., facial expressions, body movements, or cries) (3,4).

TABLE 17

General Principles for the Prevention and Management of Pain in Newborns

1. Pain in newborns is often unrecognized and undertreated. Neonates do feel pain. Compared with older age groups, newborns may experience a greater sensitivity to pain and are more susceptible to the long-term effects of painful stimulation.
2. If a procedure is painful in adults, it should be considered painful in newborns, even if they are preterm.
3. Adequate treatment of pain may be associated with decreased clinical complications and decreased mortality.
4. The appropriate use of environmental, behavioral, and pharmacologic interventions can prevent, reduce, or eliminate neonatal pain in many clinical situations.
5. Sedation does not provide pain relief and may mask the neonate's response to pain.
6. Health care professionals have the responsibility for assessment, prevention, and management of pain in neonates.

Adapted from Perkin RM, Swift JD, Raper JT. *Primer on Pediatric Palliative Care.* Greenville, NC: University Printing and Graphics of East Carolina University Press; 2005.

- Regular use of pain and other symptom assessment tools will help caregivers gauge and manage pain in the newborn (3).
- Efforts to prevent, limit, or avoid painful stimuli should occur with nonpharmacologic interventions (i.e., swaddling, positioning, nonnutritive sucking or holding with skin-to-skin contact) or appropriate medications (Table 18) (5).

TABLE 18

Medications for Neonatal Palliative Care

Drug	Category	Starting Dose (per kg body weight)	Route and Interval
Acetaminophen	Analgesic; antipyretic	24 mg load 10–15 mg 45–50 load 20–30 mg	PO once PO q4–8h PR once PR q6h
Chloral hydrate	Sedative; hypnotic	10–25 mg 25–75 mg	PO, PR q6–8h PO, PR single dose
EMLA (lidocaine-prilocaine 5%) (not to be used in neonates <37 wks' gestation)	Topical anesthetic	A thin layer of cream	Topical; 1 hr before procedure; cover with occlusive dressing
Fentanyl	Opioid analgesic	0.5–4 µg 0.5–5 µg/kg/hr	IV (or IM) q2–4h Continuous IV
Furosemide	Diuretic	1–2 mg	IV, PO, IM q12h
Glycopyrrolate	Anticholinergic; drying agent	0.01 mg	IV, PO, IM q4–8h
Lorazepam	Benzodiazepine; sedative, anxiolytic, anticonvulsant	0.05–0.1 mg	IV q4–8h
Methadone	Opioid analgesic	0.05–0.2 mg	IV, PO q12–24h
Metoclopramide	Antiemetic, promotility	0.03–0.1 mg	IV, PO, IM q8h

Drug	Category	Starting Dose (per kg body weight)	Route and Interval
Midazolam	Benzodiazepine; sedative, anxiolytic	0.05–0.15 mg 0.01–0.06 mg/kg/hr 0.3–0.5 mg	IV, IM q2–4h Continuous IV PO
Morphine	Opioid analgesic; decreases dyspnea	0.05–0.2 mg 0.2–0.5 mg 0.1–0.2 mg/kg/hr	IV, IM, q2–4h PO q4–6h IV continuous infusion
Naloxone	Opioid antagonist	0.1 mg 0.001 mg/kg/hr	IV, IM, SC, per ET, IV infusion
Sucrose, 12%–25%	Analgesic	1–2 mL	PO

ET, endotracheal tube; IV, intravenous; IM, intramuscular; PO, by mouth; PR, per rectum; SC, subcutaneous.

Modified from Toce S, Leuthner SR, Dokken D, et al. The high-risk newborn. In: Carter BS, Levetown M, eds. Palliative Care for Infants, Children, and Adolescents. Baltimore: Johns Hopkins University Press; 2004:247–272.

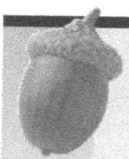

Neonatal Population
IN A NUTSHELL

Support for the parents and family are essential.

Pain control is imperative but has a number of challenges in this age group.

REFERENCES

1. American Academy of Pediatric Committee on Psychosocial Aspects of Child and Family Health. The pediatrician and childhood bereavement. Pediatrics. 1992; 89:516–518.
2. Anand KJS, Phil D and the International Evidence-Based Group for Neonatal Pain. Consensus statement for the prevention and management of pain in newborns. Arch Pediatr Adolesc Med. 2001;155:173–180.
3. Duhn LJ, Melves JM. A systematic integrative review of infant pain assessment tools. Adv Neonatol Care. 2004;4(3):126–140.
4. Buchholz M, Karl HW, Pomietto M, et al. Pain scores in infants: A modified pain scale versus visual analogue. J Pain Symptom Manage. 1998;15:117–124.
5. Toce S, Leuthner SR, Dokken D, et al. The high-risk newborn. In: Carter BS, Levetown M, eds. *Palliative Care for Infants, Children, and Adolescents*. Baltimore: Johns Hopkins University Press; 2004:247–272.

CHAPTER 92

Pediatric Intensive Care Unit

The majority of children who die do so in hospitals, most often in neonatal and pediatric intensive care units (ICUs). It is imperative that the health care team and families "use extreme responsibility, extraordinary sensitivity, and heroic compassion" (1–4).

Most children who die in an ICU do so after a decision has been made either to withhold or to withdraw life-extending therapies, including ventilators, antibiotics, intravenous fluids, and other potentially life-prolonging technologies (3–5). Here are the points to remember:

- The goal of withdrawing life-sustaining treatments is to remove unwanted treatments rather than to hasten death. It is essential in clarifying the distinction between active euthanasia (providing drugs or toxins that hasten death) and death that accompanies the withdrawal of life support.

- Withdrawing life support measures is seldom an emergency decision, and time should be taken to resolve disagreements among the staff and with the family.

- Strategies to improve consensus include allaying fears of legal liability, encouraging face-to-face discussions between health care providers who disagree on the prognosis, eliciting the views of clinicians who are providing bedside care, and consulting with a senior clinician or ethics committee.

APPROPRIATE SETTING AND MONITORING

If the child cannot be transferred to the home or to a homelike environment, the health care team should transform the ICU into a suitable place to fulfill the new goals of palliative care (Table 19). Another option is to transfer the patient from the ICU setting to a general pediatric unit or, preferably, a palliative care room. Example goals:

- Square footage large enough for family and friends to gather at the end of life of a special child

- Respite areas; indoor family space divided from patient space and outdoor seating areas

TABLE 19

Ways in Which Intensive Care Units Can Simulate a Home Environment for Dying Patients

Transportable Aspect of a Patient's Home	Ways to Provide This Aspect in the Intensive Care Unit
Privacy	Provide a private room Close doors and curtains
Ready access to family	Suspend restrictive visiting hours Provide comfortable chairs, recliners, and cots for family members in the patient's room
Access to patient's own possessions and amenities	Allow family to bring in favorite music, clothes, religious icons, food, and pets
Family serving as personal caregivers	When appropriate, allow family to assist with patient care
Access to religious rituals and spiritual support	Provide religious and spiritual resources Encourage religious and other family rituals at the bedside before and after death

Modified from Perkin RM, Swift JD, Raper JT. *Primer on Pediatric Palliative Care.* Greenville, NC: University Printing and Graphics of East Carolina University Press; 2005.

- Aesthetic environment that promotes a home environment, natural and electrical light control, and personalization areas for photos and trinkets

- Queen-size bed to promote closeness between the child, family, pets, and friends

- Window seating large enough for a parent and child; suction and oxygen capability in this area

- Kitchen area for nourishment breaks

- Technology station for communicating electronic family diary entries and for diversion activities

- Outer wall with numerous windows and a large doorway to allow the patient, family, and friends to enjoy the healing landscape and changes in the weather

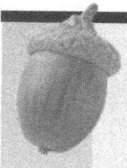

Pediatric Intensive Care Unit
IN A NUTSHELL

Palliative care in the pediatric ICU most often involves decisions regarding life support.

The goals of palliative care in the pediatric ICU involve removal of unwanted treatments rather than hastening death.

Removing life support is never an emergency, and time may be required to be sure everyone is in agreement.

The setting should be made as friendly as possible.

- Privacy fencing that allows for direct pet entry
- Home-style bathroom with a large multiple-jet shower for stress reduction
- Closet areas for patient/family storage and health care supply storage

REFERENCES

1. Wanzer SG, Federman DD, Adelstein SJ, et al. The physician's responsibility toward hopelessly ill patients: A second look. N Engl J Med. 1989;320:844–849.
2. Levetown M, Liber S, Audet M. Palliative care in the pediatric intensive care unit. In: Carter BS, Levetown M, eds. *Palliative Care for Infants, Children, and Adolescents*. Baltimore: Johns Hopkins University Press; 2004:273–291.
3. McCallum DE, Byrne P, Bruera E. How children die in hospitals. J Pain Symptom Manage. 2000;20:417–423.
4. Garros D, Rosychuk RJ, Cox PN. Circumstances surrounding end of life in a pediatric intensive care unit. Pediatrics. 2003;112:e371–e379.
5. Faber-Langendoen K, Lanken PN. Dying patients in the intensive care unit: Forgoing treatment, maintaining care. Am Intern Med. 2000;133:886–893.

CHAPTER 93

Pediatric Withdrawal of Life Support

Once an informed decision has been made by patient/family/surrogate to withdraw supportive treatment with the expectation that the patient will die, discontinuing pressors or dialysis may sometimes lead to death. More commonly, the stopping of the ventilator is the final step. This step is sometimes uncomfortable and often feared by the health care team, but it needn't be. Discontinuation of ventilatory support may be done in one of three ways: extubation, rapid weaning (few hours), or slow weaning without reversal (see Table 20). Increasingly, intensivists and pulmonologists favor extubation as the more humane approach. Whichever method is used, the steps to be taken and your expectations should be thoroughly discussed with the family. Once this has been done and an agreeable time has been set, the following guidelines may increase family and staff comfort because they are designed to maximize patient comfort:

1. **Discontinue monitors**: All monitors (IVs, oximeters, pulse, pressure, respiration, etc.) should be disconnected from the patient and/or from their power source; it is difficult to be sure that all are off; someone who knows how they operate should be present to override the alarm of any that cannot be guaranteed off (e.g., some vent alarms).

2. **Free patient's hands**: Hands are for holding; anything that restricts access to hands should be removed (restraints, mitts, bed rails, IVs, etc.).

3. **Remove encumbering and disfiguring devices**: Anything that will get in the way of the family should be removed (e.g., warming blankets, IV poles, monitors, anything stained with blood or Betadine should be removed or covered; NG tubes should be removed before the family enters the room).

4. **Invite family in**: Have tissues available in the room.

5. **The responsible physician should be present**: He or she should quietly stop the pressors and reduce the IV to KVO ("keep vein open"); IV access should be maintained.

TABLE 20

Methods of Withdrawing Ventilator Support

Method	Positive Aspects	Negative Aspects
Prolonged terminal weaning	Allows titration of drugs to control dyspnea Maintains airway for suctioning Creates more "emotional distance" between ventilator withdrawal and patient's death	May prolong the dying process May mislead family to think that survival is still a goal of therapy Interposes a machine between family and patient Precludes any possibility of verbal communication
Extubation	Allows patient to be free of unwanted technology Is less likely to prolong the dying process	Family may interpret noisy breathing caused by airway secretions or agonal breaths as discomfort May cause dyspnea at time of extubation, especially if anticipatory sedation is not given
Rapid terminal weaning	Maintains airway for suctioning Is less likely to prolong the dying process	Interposes machine between family and patient Precludes any possibility of verbal communication

From Perkin RM, Swift JD, Raper JT. *Primer on Pediatric Palliative Care.* Greenville, NC: University Printing and Graphics of East Carolina University Press; 2005.

6. **IV sedation and pain control medications should be already drawn up**: Morphine and Ativan (etc.) should be ready in case of distressing tachypnea; the family should have been made aware of agonal breathing, but if the patient appears to be in respiratory distress, he or she should be further sedated.

7. **The vent is set to F_{IO_2} of 21%**: The patient is observed for signs of respiratory distress; if the scene is comfortable the ET is removed under a clean towel; a nurse cleans the patient's face with a damp washcloth; someone is beside the vent to stop any alarm.

8. **Remain with the family**: Physician and nurse should remain in the room until death is declared; ask the family if they want some time alone with the body (1).

PLAN FOR WITHDRAWAL

- Determine which life support measures will be discontinued, in what order, and by whom.
- Redefine the goals of care in terms of patient comfort.
- The time course for withdrawal of life-sustaining treatments should equal the time to meet the child's needs for pain relief. Tapering treatments only delays death.

- Because the withdrawal of mechanical ventilation poses the greatest problems with ensuring comfort, all other life support devices should be withdrawn before the ventilator.

WITHDRAWING MECHANICAL VENTILATION

- Unless the patient specifically requests otherwise, analgesia and sedation should be provided before withdrawing mechanical ventilation support.

- Many clinicians prefer leaving the ET tube in place during withdrawal of mechanical ventilation to prevent gasping and airway occlusion that may be uncomfortable for the patient and observers. It also facilitates suctioning in patients who are uncomfortable because of profuse secretions. Nevertheless it may be appropriate to extubate the patient, particularly if the child can communicate or if prolonged survival off of life support is expected.

- Prepare the observers by reassuring them that agonal breathing is normal and part of dying.

SURVIVAL DESPITE WITHDRAWAL OF LIFE-SUSTAINING TREATMENT

- Patients may survive the withdrawal of life-sustaining treatments. Have a plan.

- Reassure the family that their child is comfortable and the timing of death is out of the control of the clinical team.

- Consider transferring these patients out of the ICU to a more private area as long as the family has been prepared for the move.

- Be wary of revising plans and prognosis based on a perceived delay in the expected timing of death. These changes in plans can have a devastating effect on family and the health care team.

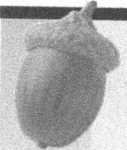

Pediatric Withdrawal of Life Support
IN A NUTSHELL

Withdrawal of life support from a pediatric patient, although similar to an adult patient, has several unique characteristics as described in the chapter.

REFERENCES

1. Perkin RM, Swift D, Raper JT, *Primer on Pediatric Palliative Care.* Greenville, NC: University Printing and Graphics of East Carolina University Press; 2005.

CHAPTER 94

The Dying Adolescent

Adolescents, especially those who are medically experienced, often demonstrate remarkable insight into their illnesses, prospects for survival, and preferences for how they wish to spend their remaining time. Research with adolescents suggests the following:

- Experience with serious medical conditions, rather than chronological age, constitutes a more reliable indicator of decision-making capability (1,2).

- When solicited in a sensitive and respectful way, many adolescents share their feelings about impending death and their opinions concerning continued treatment and palliative care (2).

- It is crucial for expressions of preference to be taken seriously by medical care providers and parents.

- The American Academy of Pediatrics (AAP) recommends that physicians respect the wishes of mature adolescents (3).

For younger adolescents who meet some but not all of the criteria for functional competence, they may be given a meaningful decisional role in which serious account is taken of their preferences but final authority rests with the responsible adult. The notion of assent rather than consent has been suggested for this population (3). This can be problematic when applied in practice. If the younger adolescent feels he or she has veto power over a recommended care plan, care providers are forced to choose between honoring a poor decision not made competently and disregarding the child's stated wish, which violates the spirit of seeking assent in the first place.

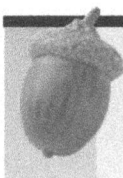

The Dying Adolescent
IN A NUTSHELL

Adolescents are often surprisingly prepared for what is happening to them.

Medical experience has more impact on decision making than does chronological age.

Expressions for preference should be taken seriously.

REFERENCES

1. Freyer DR. Care of the dying adolescent: special considerations. Pediatrics. 2004;113: 381–388.
2. Hartman RG. Dying young: cases from the courts. Arch Pediatr Adolesc Med. 2004;158: 615–619.
3. American Academy of Pediatrics, Committee on Bioethics. Informed consent, parental permission, and assent in pediatric practice. Pediatrics. 1995;95:314–317.

Charting

CHAPTER 95

Documentation in Palliative Care

The importance of documentation goes without saying, but documenting in palliative care has several unique characteristics. The idea is to **paint a picture with words**. Documentation must be **accurate and truthful**.

GENERAL

All chart documentation should follow these principles (1):

- Must be **legible** and reader friendly.
- Use **short sentences** with **one main point**.
- **Brief** is better, but cover everything that is needed.
- Record the **date and time**.
- Use approved or commonly **understood abbreviations**.
- **No liquid correction fluid**. If correction is needed, draw a line through the entry and write "error"; date and initial it. Then write a correction.

> Good documentation is like a bikini: Brief is better, but it needs to be adequate to cover the subject!

"NEGATIVE" DOCUMENTATION

Most of us in medicine were taught to document the positives in a patient's condition. The very term *progress note* implies just that—progress! However, in palliative care, **decline** is generally the rule, and documentation may, at first, seem negative. This is the **realistic picture**! Document the progressive declines by identifying the activities of daily living the patient can no longer perform or actively participate in, as compared to last week, last month, and so on.

Some of the most important facts to document include the following:

- **Mental status**: Awake (this is different than alert!), lethargic; hard to arouse; responsive to verbal stimuli and/or responsive to touch
- **Weight loss**: Compared to baseline (usual body weight)
- **Functional decline**: General
- **Cognitive decline**: Orientation to person, place, and time, level of confusion, memory loss, and attention span
- Dependence on **ADLs (see Table 21 for a helpful mnemonic)**
  - **Dressing**: Level of assistance required
  - **Eating**: Does patient need cueing to eat or needs to be fed; type of diet; percentage of diet taken; supplements
  - **Ambulation**: Can the patient transfer; is a lift needed; does the patient use assistive devices; wheelchair bound; can they self-propel the wheelchair
  - **Toileting**: Incontinence of bowel and bladder
  - **Hygiene**: Assistance needed with bathing
- **Ability to speak**: Is speech understandable; "word salad"; difficulty with "word finding." Can patient use sentences or speak more than six words?
- **Muscle wasting** or cachexia
- **Color**: Pale, jaundice, ashen, cyanotic

COMPARE TO A "NORMAL" PERSON

A palliative patient may be "doing fine" when compared to his or her previous condition but may still be anorexic, totally confused, and dependent on staff for all ADLs. When charting, **compare to a normal**, fully active and productive individual. When reviewers see "doing well" or "having a good day" on the chart, they think the patient is ready to return to the work force!

TABLE 21

Mnemonics

IADLs	ADLs
Independent Activities of Daily Living	Activities of Daily Living
(Lose these and you get the SHAFT.)	(Lose these and you are nearing the end of life.)
S—Shopping	D—Dressing
H—Housekeeping	E—Eating
A—Accounting (checkbook)	A—Ambulation
F—Food preparation	T—Toileting
T—Travel	H—Hygiene (bathing)

LANGUAGE

Common words used to describe palliative patients may be very helpful in "painting the picture with words."

- "Slumped over in chair."
- "Found with head resting on chest."
- "Unable to walk more than 6 feet."
- "Not tracking visually."
- "Drooling"
- "Blank stare"
- "No response to . . . loud noise . . . squeezing of hand . . . calling of name"
- Document reality: "The patient is dying."

For symptoms of the end stages of various disease processes, see Tables 22 through 28.

TABLE 22

Debility/Failure to Thrive

Subjective	Objective
Disorientated	Weight loss
Dependent on staff for all ADLs	Lethargy
Assistance with dressing	Somnolence
Assistance with bathing	Disoriented
Incontinent of bowel and bladder	Garbled speech
Unsteady gait	Unintelligible speech
Retropulsion	Word salad
Fall risk	Limited speech pattern
Nonambulatory	Inappropriate speech pattern
Wheelchair bound	Cachectic
Unable to self-propel wheelchair	Lost ability to smile
Bedbound	Atrophy of facial muscles
Requires lift to transfer	Muscle wasting
Fetal position	Flat affect
Decreased appetite	Fragile skin integrity
Pocketing food	Muscle wasting
Requires hand feeding	Erythema over pressure points
Requires cueing to eat	Contractures
Eats—%	Combative
Requires pureed diet	Unable to hold head up without assistive
Requires thickened liquids	device
Frequent choking	Slumped forward in wheelchair
Aspiration	Drooling

(continued)

TABLE 22 (Continued)

Debility/Failure to Thrive

Subjective	Objective
Lethargic	Fetal position
Sleeps most of the day	Agitation
Unable to make needs known	Pressure ulcers
Refuses medications	Protective devices in place

TABLE 23

End-Stage Dementia

Subjective	Objective
10% weight loss in last 6 months	Weight loss
Pneumonia	Cachectic
Upper UTI	Frail
Infected stage 3 or 4 wounds	Pale
Disorientated	Appearing older than known age
Dependent on staff for all ADLs	Uncooperative with exam
Assistance with dressing	Combative
Assistance with bathing	Lethargy
Lost ability to smile	Somnolence
Incontinent of bowel and bladder	Disoriented
Unsteady gait	Garbled speech
Retropulsion	Unintelligible speech
Fall risk	Word salad
Nonambulatory	Limited speech pattern
Wheelchair bound	Inappropriate speech pattern
Unable to self-propel wheelchair	Lost ability to smile
Bedbound	Atrophy of facial muscles
Requires lift to transfer	Muscle wasting
Fetal position	Flat affect
Decreased appetite	Blank stare
Pocketing food	Fragile skin integrity
Requires hand feeding	Muscle atrophy
Requires cueing to eat	Erythema over pressure points
Eats—%	Contractures
Requires pureed diet	Unable to hold head up without assistive device
Requires thickened liquids	
Dysphagia	Slumped forward in wheelchair
Frequent choking	Drooling
Aspiration	Fetal position
Lethargic	Agitation

Subjective	Objective
Sleeps most of the day	Pressure ulcers
Unable to make needs known	Protective devices in place
Refuses medications	Edema
Progressive decline	Limited range of motion

TABLE 24

End-Stage Cardiac Disease

Subjective	Objective
Chest pain	Tachycardia
Angina	Bradycardia
Dyspnea at rest	Irregular pulse
Dyspnea with exertion	Hypotension
Dyspnea during conversation	Cyanosis
Dyspnea while eating	Pale
Oxygen dependent	Diaphoresis
Refuses oxygen	Jugular venous distention
Orthopnea	Carotid bruit
Paroxysmal nocturnal dyspnea	Diminished breath sounds
Cough: dry/productive	Wet rales
Severe fatigue	Wheezing
Weakness	Pleural effusion
Lethargy	Cardiac murmur
Somnolence	Hepatomegaly
Palpitations	Ascites
Weight gain/loss	Pitting edema
Syncope	Changes of long-standing pedal edema
Uses two or three pillows	Peripheral vascular disease
Cannot walk more than_____	Distal ischemia

TABLE 25

End-Stage Renal Disease

Subjective	Objective
Decreased urine output	Disorientation
Oliguria	Ashen color
Anuria	Pale
Intractable nausea and vomiting	Cachetic
Confusion	Muscle wasting

(continued)

TABLE 25 (Continued)

End-Stage Renal Disease

Subjective	Objective
Restlessness	Puffy
Agitation	Edema
Disorientation	Increased skin turgor
Hallucinations	Periorbital edema
Obtunded	Jaundice
Unresponsive to verbal stimuli	Jugular venous distention
Unable to make needs known	Irregular pulse
Decreased ambulatory status	Cardiac murmur
Bedbound	Tachycardia
Wheelchair bound	Bradycardia
Lift transfers	Ascites
Incontinent	Hepatomegaly
Requires assistance with ADLs	Petechia
Depression	Ecchymosis
Itching	Decreased skin integrity
History of sepsis	Wet rales
History of hypoglycemia	Albumin <3.5 g/dL
History of pneumonia	Co-morbidities of_____
History of pyelonephritis	Hyperkalemia: potassium >7.0
Uremic pericarditis	Serum creatinine >8 mg/dL
Diabetic	Creatinine clearance <10 mL/min
Immunosuppression	Platelet <25,000

TABLE 26

End-Stage Pulmonary Disease

Subjective	Objective
Disabling dyspnea at rest	Disorientation
Dyspnea on exertion	Cyanosis
Dyspnea during conversation	Dusky
Dyspnea while eating	Cushinoid appearance
Walking distance of_____	Weight loss
Oxygen dependent	Using accessory muscles
Refuses supplemental oxygen	Pursed lip breathing
Weakness	Leans forward to breath
Extreme fatigue	Barrel chest
Homebound	Increased anterior-posterior diameter of
Chairbound	chest
Wheelchair dependent for distances	Jugular venous distention
Bed-to-chair existence	Increased expiratory phase
Bedbound	Wheezing

Subjective	Objective
Air hunger	Rhonchi
Chest pressure	Rales
Chest pain	Pulmonary congestion
Angina	Diminished breath sounds
Orthopnea	Distant heart sounds
Increased sputum	Tachycardia at rest >100/min
Cough: productive	Clubbing
Cor pulmonale	Edema
>ER/hospital visits	FEV_1 (forced expiratory volume in 1 second) <30%
	Oxygen saturation levels <88%

TABLE 27

End-Stage Liver Disease

Subjective	Objective
Disorientation	Disorientation
Confusion	Deliberate speech
Hallucinations	Garbled speech
Fatigue	Unintelligible speech
Weakness	Jaundiced
Obtunded	Pale
Lethargy	Cachetic
Somnolence	Muscle wasting
Unresponsive to verbal stimuli	Increased skin turgor
Unable to make needs known	Periorbital edema
Intractable nausea and vomiting	Jugular venous distention
Restlessness	Irregular cardiac rhythm
Agitation	Cardiac murmur
Combative	Tachycardia
Decreased ambulatory status	Bradycardia
Bed-to-chair existence	Ascites
Bedbound	Abdominal girth
Wheelchair bound	Fluid wave
Lift transfers	Distant bowel sounds
Incontinent bowel and bladder	Edema
Requires assistance with ADLs	Hepatomegaly
Depression	Petechia
Itching	Ecchymosis
History of pneumonia	Decreased skin integrity
Immunosuppression	Dupuytren's contractures
Alcohol intake	Palmar erythema
Weight loss	Albumin <2.5 g/dL

TABLE 28

End-Stage Neurologic Disease and Cerebrovascular Accident

Subjective	Objective
Dependent on staff for all ADLs	Disoriented
Assistance with dressing	Combative
Assistance with bathing	Lethargy
Lost ability to smile	Somnolence
Incontinent of bowel and bladder	Unresponsive to verbal stimuli
Unsteady gait	Unresponsive to touch
Retropulsion	Garbled speech
Fall risk	Unintelligible speech
Shuffling gait	Word salad
Paraplegia	Limited speech pattern
Nonambulatory	Inappropriate speech pattern
Wheelchair bound	Nonverbal
Unable to self-propel wheelchair	Uncooperative with exam
Bedbound	Combative
Requires lift to transfer	Weight loss
Fetal position	Cachectic
Decreased appetite	Frail
Pocketing food	Pale
Requires hand feeding	Appearing older than known age
Requires cueing to eat	Lost ability to smile
Eats_____%	Facial asymmetry
Requires pureed diet	Atrophy of facial muscles
Requires thickened liquids	Muscle wasting
Finger foods	Flat affect
Soft diet	Blank stare
Frequent choking	Doll's eyes
Aspiration	Pupils fixed
Inability to clear secretions	Fragile skin integrity
Dysphagia	Muscle atrophy
Lethargic	Erythema over pressure points
Sleeps most of the day	Contractures
Unable to make needs known	Unable to hold head up without assistive
Refuses medications	device
Progressive decline	Slumped forward in wheelchair
10% weight loss in last 6 months	Drooling
Pneumonia	Fetal position
Upper urinary tract infection	Agitation
Infected stage 3 or 4 wounds	Pressure ulcers
Sepsis	Protective devices in place
Palliative Performance Scale <50%	Edema
Bed rails	Limited range of motion

Subjective	Objective
Low air loss mattress	Tremors
	Foot drop
	Ataxia

INTERDISCIPLINARY CARE

Good end-of-life care involves an **interdisciplinary** approach with physicians, nurses, aides, social workers, chaplains, and others documenting on the chart. Good documentation involves:

- **Reading** the other discipline's notes
- Writing notes that **do not contradict** the other disciplines. If you don't agree, talk to the other disciplines and decide on a plan of action. A patient's chart is not the place to question or degrade someone else!
- **Share information:** "Social worker or chaplain reports spiritual pain."
- Develop a single set of **goals**, with treatment and alternatives clearly documented so the patient and family can make informed choices (2).

ACTION

Describe who you talked to and what action was taken or what recommendations were given. The documentation should "stand on its own" (3):

- Document the patient's **expected outcomes** (realistic!)
- Document the **interventions** implemented.
- Document the patient's **response** to the interventions.

REFERENCES

1. Hospice and Palliative Nurses Association. *Core Curriculum for the Generalist Hospice and Palliative Nurse*. Dubuque, Iowa: Kendall/Hunt; 2005.
2. *Clinical Practice Guidelines for Quality Palliative Care*. Pittsburgh: National Consensus Project for Quality Palliative Care; 2004.
3. *Mosby's Surefire Documentation: How, What and When Nurses Need to Document*. 2nd ed. Philadelphia: Mosby, Elsevier Health Science; 2006.

CHAPTER 96

Coding and Billing for Hospice/Palliative Care

According to the Health Care Financing Administration and American Medical Association's CPT Information Services, "There are no specific CPT codes for evaluation and management services provided by a physician to a patient receiving hospice care in any location. When a Medicare beneficiary elects the hospice benefit, Medicare pays the hospice for all services related to the terminal illness through four set per diem rates. The exception to this is physician services."

Medicare hospice regulations, at 42 CFR 418.304(c), state that services of the patient's attending physician, who is not employed by the hospice or providing services under arrangements with the hospice, are not considered hospice services. These services are billed directly to Medicare Part B according to procedures established in 42 CFR 405 subparts D and E. When provided by an attending physician, as just described, evaluation and management services provided to hospice patients would be billed in the following manner:

- If the evaluation and management services are provided to a hospice patient who is residing in a nursing facility, then the subsequent nursing facility care codes are billed (99301–99316 series).

- If the evaluation and management services are provided to a hospice patient in their private residence, the home service codes are billed (99341–99350 series). The physician must provide the evaluation and management services in the patient's home in order for these codes to be billed.

- If the evaluation and management services are provided to a patient in a board and care type facility, including a hospice residential facility, then domiciliary/rest home codes are billed (99321–99333 series). Again, these services must be provided in the facility in order for the domiciliary/rest home codes to be billed.

If another physician covers for the attending physician, the attending physician must bill Medicare Part B for the services using either the Q5 or Q6 modifier, in addition to the GV or GW modifier. Use the Q5 modifier for service furnished by a substitute physician under a reciprocal billing arrangement. Use the Q6 modifier for service furnished by a *locum tenens* (substitute) physician. The GV modifier indicates the

Billing Hospice Physician Services (Related to Terminal Diagnosis)

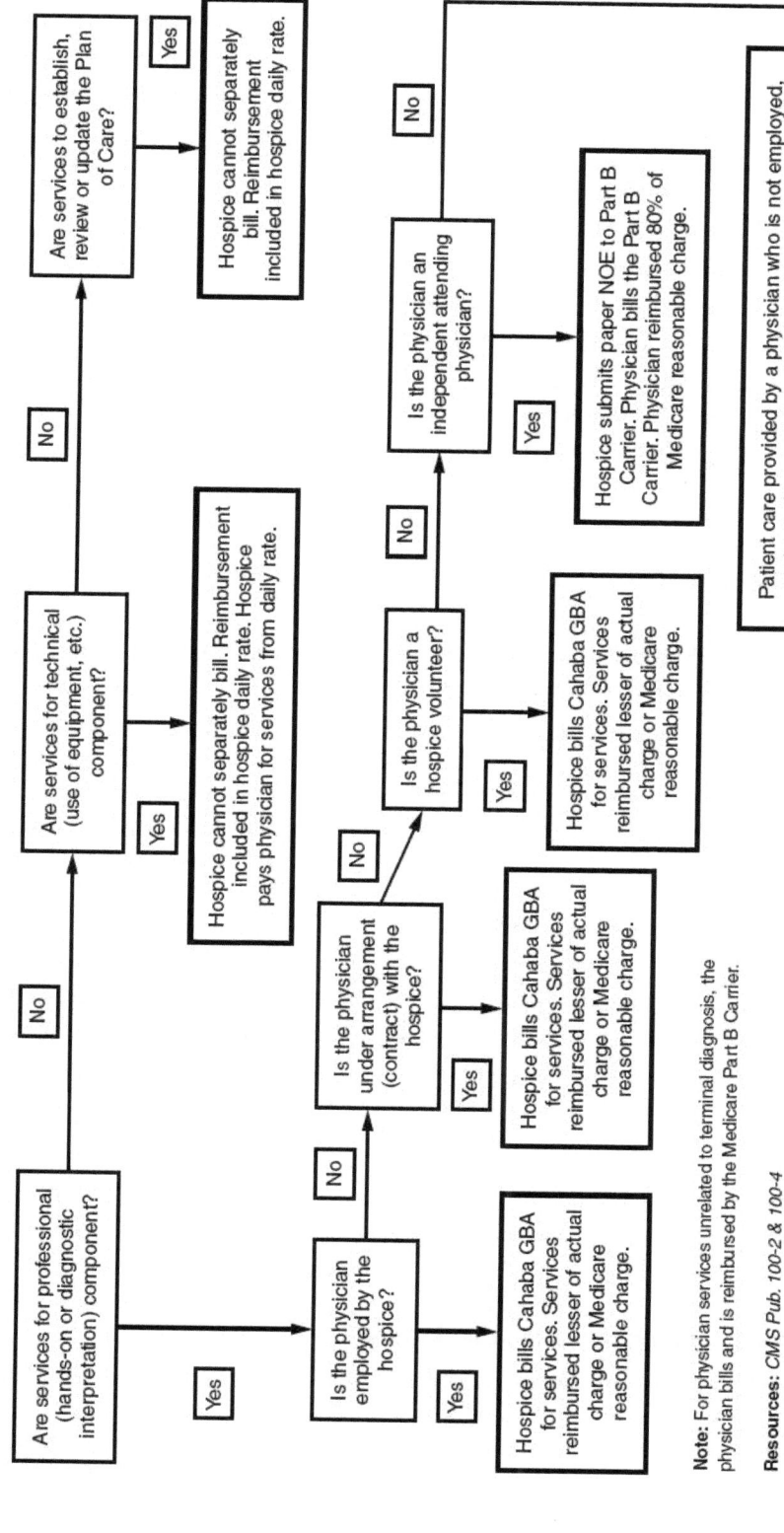

Note: For physician services unrelated to terminal diagnosis, the physician bills and is reimbursed by the Medicare Part B Carrier.

Resources: *CMS Pub. 100-2 & 100-4*
Claims Filing & Coverage Guidelines section of MRG
Cahaba GBA
A CMS Contracted Intermediary
November 2003

FIGURE 11 ◉ Billing hospice physician services related to terminal diagnosis.

service was related to the terminal illness, whereas the GW modifier indicates the service was not related to the terminal illness (Figure 11).

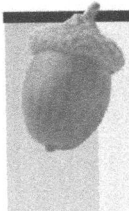

Hospice Billing
IN A NUTSHELL

Patients can continue to receive care from their attending physician for all illnesses related and unrelated to the terminal diagnosis.

Independent attending physician continues to bill Medicare Part B as before using same ICD-9 and CPT codes

If an associate sees the patient, the attending physician of record must bill Medicare Part B for the services using either the Q5 or Q6 modifier, in addition to the GV or GW modifier.

FREQUENTLY ASKED QUESTIONS ABOUT THE MEDICARE HOSPICE BENEFIT (SUPPLEMENTAL)

How can you tell when a patient has 6 months or less to live in order to qualify for the Medicare hospice benefit?

The Centers for Medicare & Medicaid Services (CMS) have developed guidelines for establishing a 6-month prognosis for several noncancer terminal illnesses. Those guidelines (see appendix), as contained in this booklet, are based on normal disease progression. If a patient's disease process does not run a "normal course," the benefits can be extended through recertification.

What are hospice benefit periods?

In the past, there were four benefit periods, (90, 60, 30 days, then a fourth period that was unlimited). Many patients had entered their 4th benefit period and were in fear of losing their hospice benefits if they were to remain on hospice until they died. Since the end of 1997, the benefit periods have been revised. Now the patient has 90-, 90-, then continuous 60-day benefit periods for physician recertification of terminality. For example, if a patient improves and is not felt to be terminal at the end of the 2nd benefit period, then the patient can come off hospice care and be restarted when the patient's prognosis worsens again. For the initial 90-day benefit period, both the hospice medical director and the patient's attending physician must certify the patient. For all subsequent benefit periods, recertification is only required from the hospice medical director.

How is the attending physician reimbursed?

Attending physicians who are *not employed by the hospice* continue to bill *Medicare* for their services with the same ICD-9 and CPT codes they have previously used. If the physician *is employed by the hospice* caring for that patient, the *hospice* is billed for the level of service provided. If the physician is salaried by a *different hospice* and not by the hospice caring for the patient, *Medicare* is billed for the level of service provided. If an associate sees the patient, the attending physician of record must bill Medicare Part B for the services using either the Q5 or Q6 modifier, in addition to the GV or GW modifier. HCFA receives a record of the name of each attending physician for each hospice patient.

Can a nurse practitioner serve as an attending physician?

Section 408 of the Medicare Prescription Drug Improvement and Modernization Act of 2003 (MMA) amended the Social Security Act (Section 1861[dd][3][B]) and Section 1814(a)(7) to include nurse practitioners in the definition of an attending physician for hospice beneficiaries. Beginning December 8, 2003, Medicare pays for services, with the exception of certifying the terminal illness with a prognosis of 6 months or less, provided by nurse practitioners to Medicare beneficiaries who have selected a nurse practitioner as their attending physician. A physician will be required to certify the terminal illness and 6-month prognosis.

REFERENCES

1. National Hospice and Palliative Care Organization statistics. Available at: www.nhpco.org/nds.
2. Centers for Medicare & Medicaid Services. Hospice Center. Available at: http://www.cms .hhs.gov/center/hospice.asp. Accessed July 9, 2006.

Ethics at the
End of Life

CHAPTER 97

Ethics and Legal Issues

Legal precedent is often set by **previous cases**. Because many ethical issues in end-of-life care are **relatively new**, secondary to rapid advances in modern medicine, specific legal parameters are often lacking. The biggest legal issues that come up in the area of ethics at end of life usually involve **hastening of death** and **advanced directives**.

HASTENED DEATH

Legally and ethically, hastening someone's death usually involves the **rule of double effect** (see Chapter 98):

- **Intent** of the treatment is paramount in both legal and ethical areas (1): If the intent is to help the patient (e.g., a risky surgery or separating Siamese twins when one may die, to save the other), there are generally no legal ramifications. But in America, you can be sued for anything!

- Clinicians may legally administer **potentially lethal medications** when necessary to relieve a terminally ill patient's suffering (2).

- Assisted suicide remains controversial. However there has been a general refusal of jurors to convict physicians contributing to the consensual deaths of terminally ill patients.

- Western law and culture favors **full disclosure** and **patient autonomy** over the protection offered by others.

ADVANCED DIRECTIVES

Health care providers are **legally obligated** (Patient Self-determination Act, 1991) to follow a patient's advanced directive. However, they often do not (3). Important legal points to remember about advanced directives include the following:

- No advanced directive is in effect as long as the patient is **decisional**.

- A decisional patient has the right to make stupid (bad) decisions.

- The **law requires** clinicians to forgo treatment at the request of a decisional patient, even if that decision will lead to the patient's death (removing life support from a decisional patient).

- **Terminal sedation** with the patient's informed consent is legal.

- Patients may **refuse** any medical intervention—treating decisional patients against their will is seen legally as violating their physical integrity (battery) (1).

- Clinicians often do not know the patient's wishes or whether or not the patient has an advanced directive (4).

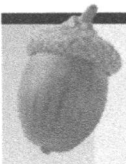

Ethics and Legal Issues
IN A NUTSHELL

Intent to follow the patient's **goals** is the basis for most ethical and legal decisions in end of life.

Advanced directives are legally and ethically binding: Patient autonomy is favored in Western law.

REFERENCES

1. Quill TE, Dresser R, Brock DW. The rule of double effect—a critique of its role in end-of-life decision making. N Engl J Med. 1997;337:1768–1771.
2. Cantor NL, Thomas GC. Pain relief, acceleration of death, and criminal law. Kennedy Inst Ethics J. 1996;6:107–127.
3. Warm E. Eight myths about advance directives. *Fast Facts and Concepts #12*. Milwaukee: Medical College of Wisconsin; 2002.
4. The SUPPORT Principal Investigators. A controlled trial to improve care for seriously ill hospitalized patients: the study to understand prognoses and preferences for outcomes and risks of treatments (SUPPORT) [published correction appears in JAMA. 1996;275:1232]. JAMA. 1995;274:1591–1598.

CHAPTER 98

Hastened Death: The Rule of Double Effect

The **rule of double effect** became part of Roman Catholic thought in the Middle Ages and was applied to situations where a person **could not avoid all harmful outcomes** (1). It is an ethical principle used in palliative medicine today but also **applies to most situations in medicine**.

For example, a patient suffering with severe pain from a dissecting abdominal aortic aneurysm has only poor options. The person may choose surgery and not survive. Ethically, however, the surgery did not kill the patient because the intent was to help. This applies to palliative care as well. Pain medications, palliative procedures, and palliative sedation are all intended to help relieve suffering. If the **intent** is to help the patient, even if one of those treatments does hasten death, it is ethically appropriate. If the **intent** is to harm the patient, then it is considered unethical by this principle.

CLINICAL APPLICATIONS

The rule of double effect does not cover all clinical situations, but it can be helpful. Here are the main points:

- When offering a medical therapy, the **intent** of that therapy determines if it is ethical.

- All medical treatments have both intended and unintended effects.

- The clinical scenario in giving morphine to relieve pain, even if it may hasten the patient's death, is largely overemphasized. Morphine's risk of adverse side effects, including respiratory depression, is vastly overestimated (2).

- **Ethics** at end of life are often **guided by the patient's goals**. Once the goals are known, treatment (or lack of treatments) often becomes clear.

- The degree of suffering, informed consent, and the absence of less harmful alternative treatment should all be considered (3).

Remember: The *disease* is killing the patient not the treatment!

"I don't want to be the last one to give the medication."
Remember: Someone is going to give the last everything—gelatin, haircut, and so on. Isn't it a privilege to be the last to help the patient be comfortable?

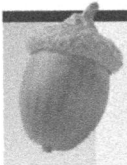

Hastened Death: The Rule of Double Effect
IN A NUTSHELL

If the **intent** is to help the patient and the potential outcome is good (such as relieving pain) but a potentially bad side effect exists (death), that treatment is considered ethical.

REFERENCES

1. Pope John Paul II. *Evangelium vitae*. Washington, DC: U.S. Catholic Conference, March 30, 1995:189.
2. Emanuel LL, von Gunten CF, Ferris FD. *The Education for Physicians on End-of-Life Care (EPEC) Curriculum*. Chicago: American Medical Association; 1999.
3. Quill TE, Dresser R, Brock DW. The rule of double effect—a critique of its role in end-of-life decision making. N Engl J Med. 1997;337:1768–1771.

CHAPTER 99

When to Stop—Medical Futility

Our society is beginning to recognize the scientific **limitations of modern medicine** and that some treatments offer **no real hope or benefit to the patient** (1). Indeed, they may be causing harm.

NONBENEFICIAL TREATMENTS

Ethically, these statements are **generally accepted** at this time (2–4):

- Just because a medical therapy exists, it **does not have to be used**.
- **All patients eventually die**, regardless of therapies.
- A decisional adult has the **right to refuse** medical therapy, even life-sustaining treatments.
- **Doing everything** possible to sustain life is **not always beneficial** to the patient.
- Medical decisions should be made by **balancing** the **potential benefits and burdens**.
- **Quality of life** is a factor in accepting or not accepting life prolonging therapies.
- **Advanced directives**, or the patient's known wishes, **should be honored** when the patient is not decisional.
- Ethically, **withholding or withdrawing** life prolonging therapies are the **same**: Both allow the disease to progress on its natural course.

> Once a patient's *goals* are determined, ethical issues often fall into place.

REASONS TO STOP

Ethically there are **three "reasonable" times** to withhold or stop life support (5–7):

1. **It's not going to work**: This is like CPR on dead people (See Table 29. The public doesn't understand the limitations of CPR!) This is the easiest decision to make because the patient makes it for you!

TABLE 29

Effectiveness of CPR

- **In-hospital CPR: 15.2% survival rate to discharge** worldwide
- (United States, 15%; Canada, 16%; UK, 17%; other European countries, 14%):
    - **Chest wall trauma: 75%.**
    - **Aspiration: 25%–50%.**
- **Long-term care survival:**
    - Of 115 patients, 95 were dead on arrival; other 10 died in 48 hours.
    - Other studies: 0%–5%.

Sources: Saklayen M, Liss H, Market R. In-hospital cardiopulmonology resuscitation: survival in one hospital and literature review. Medicine (Baltimore). 1995;74:163–175. Long-term care survival statistics presented at the American Academy of Hospice and Palliative Medicine Conference, 2004.

2. We might drag a little more time out of the clock, but **we won't like what we have**: quality of life issues, permanent vegetative state, and so on.

3. We **already don't like what we have**: Penicillin may cure the pneumonia, but we may welcome the opportunistic infection in the patient with end-stage dementia!

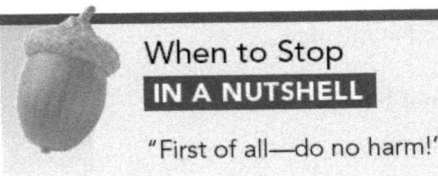

When to Stop
IN A NUTSHELL

"First of all—do no harm!"

REFERENCES

1. Storey P, Knight CF. *Ethical and Legal Decision Making When Caring for the Terminally Ill.* UNIPAC Six. Glenview, Ill: American Academy of Hospice and Palliative Medicine, 2003:43.
2. Finucance TE, Harper M. Ethical decision-making near the end of life. Clin Geriatr Med. 1996;12:369–377.
3. EPEC Project. *Withholding, Withdrawing Therapy.* Module 11. Institute for Ethics at the American Medical Association; 1999.
4. Henig NR, Faul JL, Raffin TA. Biomedical ethics and the withdrawal of advanced life support. Annu Rev Med. 2001;52:79–92.
5. Dickenson DL. Are medical ethicists out of touch? Practitioner attitudes in the US and UK towards decisions at the end-of-life. J Med Ethics. 2000;26:254–260.
6. Quill TE, Dresser R, Brock DW. The rule of double effect—a critique of its role in end-of-life decision making. N Engl J Med. 1997;337:1768–1771.
7. Victoroff MS. Ethical issues. Paper presented at: Geriatric Medicine for the Family Physician Conference; October 17, 2003; Monterey, Calif.

CHAPTER 100

Caring for Yourself and Avoiding Burnout

Palliative care is **unique** because of how closely we work with the patient and family to identify the goals, values, preferences, and needs throughout the illness trajectory to death. **Good clinicians reject disengagement** and allow themselves to feel the **normal human emotions** associated with the process of dying. However, we must not let **unexamined emotion** interfere with our task of caring for our patients or lead to burnout.

SELF-AWARENESS

Anyone working with end-of-life issues must **examine themselves** and become aware of their own feelings on mortality. Self-awareness includes the following:

- Am I able to **say no**?
- Can I separate my **work and personal life**?
- Do I think I can **solve other people's problems**?
- Do people become easily **dependent on me**?
- How do I react to increased demands—is it to **work harder**?
- Can I **set boundaries**?

RISK FACTORS

A **well balanced clinician** is aware of certain patients and situations that are more difficult (1):

- Patient with **similar** profession, age, appearance, and so on.
- **Close relationship**—family member, friend.
- **Disagreement** with family about medical goals.
- **Children**
- Situation where there is a feeling of **failure or inadequacy**.

SIGNS AND SYMPTOMS

These are the common signs and symptoms leading to professional burnout (2). Many times the people involved are so busy they don't recognize these symptoms; we must therefore be aware of them in our **colleagues**:

- Caregiving is **no longer fun or rewarding**.
- **Emotional exhaustion**.
- **Depersonalization**.
- Diminished feelings of **personal accomplishment**.
- **Avoiding** the patient or family—or more frequent contact with the patient or family than is medically necessary.
- Sense of **self-blame, failure, guilt**.
- Physical signs of **stress**.

TREATMENT

Deep emotions for the health care provider dealing with end of life are **normal and inevitable**. Therefore, they do not need to be treated as a **disorder**, but they need to be **acknowledged and understood**. Here are some of the proven approaches (3):

- **Naming the feeling**: Once the feeling is recognized, it is much easier to deal with.
- Accept the **normalcy** of the feeling.
- Reflect on the **consequences** of the feelings.
- Consult a trusted **colleague** to reduce isolation and build a network of support.

> "You know you are an addictive rescuer when you are drowning and someone else's life flashes before your eyes."—Ben Wolfe, MEd, LCSW

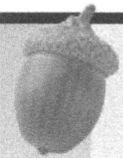

Caring for Self and Avoiding Burnout
IN A NUTSHELL

Be **aware** of your limits and boundaries.

Watch out for situations and patients that are "**high risk**."

Recognize signs and symptoms of burnout and unexamined emotions, in yourself as well as colleagues.

Name the emotion and treat it before it leads to impairment.

REFERENCES

1. Marshall AA, Smith RC. Physicians' emotional reaction to patients: recognizing and managing countertransference. Am J Gastroenterol. 1995;90:4–8.
2. Maslach C, Jackson SE, Leiter MP. Job burnout. Annu Rev Psychol. 2001;52:397–422.
3. Meier DE, Back AL, Morrison RS. The inner life of physicians and care of the seriously ill. JAMA. 2001;286:3007–3014.

Appendix Contents

1. Medications for Neonatal/Pediatric Palliative Care
2. Equianalgesic Dosing Chart
3. The Wilda Assessment
4. Analgesic Ladder
5. Principles of Pain Management
6. Opioid Conversion Examples
7. Adjuvants to Opioid Therapy
8. Medical Guidelines for Specific Diseases
    - End Stage Dementia
    - End Stage Heart Disease
    - End Stage HIV Disease
    - End Stage Liver Disease
    - End Stage Pulmonary Disease
    - End Stage Renal Disease
    - End Stage Stroke and Coma
    - General Debility
    - Amyotrophic Lateral Sclerosis (ALS)
9. Functional Assessment Staging (FAST Scale)
10. Palliative Performance Scale (PPS)
11. Weight Chart for Women
12. Weight Chart for Men
13. Calculating Your Frame Size
14. Weight Table for Women 65 and Older
15. Weight Table for Men Aged 65 and Older
16. Stages of Heart Disease

Medications for Neonatal/ Pediatric Palliative Care

Drug	Category	Starting dose (per kg body weight)	Route and interval
Acetaminophen	Analgesic, antipyretic	24 mg load 10–15 mg 45–50 load 20–30 mg	PO once PO every 4–8 hrs PR once PR every 6 hrs
Chloral hydrate	Sedative, hypnotic	10–25 mg 25–75 mg	PO, PR every 6–8 hrs PO, PR single dose
EMLA (lidocaine-prilocaine 5%) – not to be used in neonates <37 weeks gestation	Topical anesthetic	A thin layer of cream	Topical, 1 hour before procedure; cover with occlusive dressing
Fentanyl	Opioid analgesic	0.5–4 mcg 0.5–5 mcg/kg/hr	IV (or IM) every 2–4 hrs Continuous IV
Furosemide	Diuretic	1–2 mg	IV, PO, IM every 12 hrs
Glycopyrrolate	Anticholinergic drying agent	0.01 mg	IV, PO, IM every 4–8 hrs
Lorazepam	Benzodiazepine Sedative, Anxiolytic, Anticonvulsant	0.05–0.1 mg	IV every 4–8 hrs
Methadone	Opioid analgesic	0.05–0.2 mg	IV, PO every 12–24 hrs
Metoclopramide	Antiemetic, Promotility	0.03–0.1 mg	IV, PO, IM every 8 hrs
Midazolam	Benzodiazepine Sedative, Anxiolytic	0.05–0.15 mg 0.01–0.06 mg/kg/hr 0.3–0.5 mg	IV, IM every 2–4 hrs Continuous IV PO
Morphine	Opioid analgesic, Decreases dyspnea	0.05–0.2 mg 0.2–0.5 mg 0.1–0.2 mg/kg/hr	IV, IM, every 2–4 hrs PO every 4–6 hrs IV continuous infusion
Naloxone	Opioid antagonist	0.1 mg 0.001 mg/kg/hr	IV, IM, SC, per ET IV infusion
Sucrose 12–25%	Analgesic	1–2 ml	PO

APPENDIX 2

Equianalgesic Dosing Chart

Opioid	Selected Forms Available	Equianalgesic Dose	Dose Interval	Comments
Short Acting				
Morphine	**Tablets**—MSIR: 15; 30 mg	PO/PR: 30 mg	2–4 hours	May cause systemic vasodilatation due to histamine release.
	Liquid—Roxanol Concentrate: 20 mg/mL		2–4 hrs	
	Suppository—Rectal Morphine Sulfate 5, 10, 20, 30 mg	IV, SQ: 10 mg		Roxanol-T is colored orange and has a fruit taste; Regular Roxanol is clear and has an unpleasant taste
Hydromorphone	**Tablets**—Dilaudid: 1, 2, 4, 8 mg	PO/PR: 7.5 mg	2–4 hrs	The 8 mg tablet is scored.
	Liquid—Dilaudid: 1 mg/mL			
	Suppository—Dilaudid: 3 mg	IV: 1.5 mg	2–4 hrs	
Oxycodone	**Tablets**—OxyIR or Roxicodone: 5, 15, 30 mg Oxycodone/ Acetaminophine: Percocet: 2.5/325, 5/325, 7.5/325/ 10/325 Roxicet: 5/325, Tylox 5/500 mg Oxycodone/Aspirin: Percodan: 2.5/325, 5/325 mg **Liquid**—Roxicodone: 1 mg/mL, 20 mg/mL; OxyFAST: 20 mg/mL	PO: 20–30 mg	2–4 hrs	Maximum daily dose of combination oxycodone/ acetaminophen products limited by maximum acetaminophen daily dose of 4000 mg (less in the elderly or with liver failure)
Fentanyl	**Oral Transmucosal** Actiq: 200, 400, 600, 800, 1200, 1600 mcg	IV: 100 mcg OTFC: Unknown	30–60 min 30–60 min	Opioid of choice for patients with renal or liver disease. Onset OTFC is 5 min. OTFC should not be used in opiate-naïve patients

Hydrocodone	**Tablets—** **Hydrocodone/** **Acetaminophen:** Lortab: 2.5/500, 5/500, 7.5/500 10/500 mg Lorcet: 10/650 mg Norco: 5/325, 7.5/325, 10/325 mg Vicodin: 5/500, ES 7.5/750, HP 10/660 mg **Hydrocodone/** **Ibuprofen:** Vicoprofen: 7.5/200 mg **Liquid—** **Hydrocodone/** **Acetaminophen:** Lortab Elixer: 7.5/500 mg per 15 mL	PO: 30 mg	3–4 hrs	Only available in combination products that include acetaminophen or ibuprofen. Maximum dose is limited by these products. (4000 mg/24 hrs. Acetaminophen— less in elderly or liver disease; Consider side effects of ibuprofen)
Meperdine	**Tablets**—Demerol: 50, 100 mg **Liquid**—Demerol: 10 mg/mL	PO 300 mg IV 75 mg	PO Not Recom- mended 2–3 hrs	Contraindicated in renal disease. **Not for chronic pain.** Active metabolite causes CNS excitation and seizures. Max dose 600 mg/24 hrs

Long Acting

Morphine	**Tablets—** Ms Contin 15, 30, 60, 100, 200 mg Oramorph SR 15, 30, 60, 100 mg Avinza: 30, 60, 90, 120 mg Kadian 20, 30, 50, 60, 100 mg	PO 30 mg	8–12 hrs 24 hrs	Kadian and Avinza are capsules that may be opened and poured down a G tube.
Oxycodone	**Tablets**—Oxycontin 10, 20, 40, 80	PO 30 mg	8–12 hrs	Sustained release tablet—do not cut or crush
Fentanyl	**Transdermal patch—** 12, 25, 50, 75, 100 mcg/hr	TD 15 mcg	72 hrs	Onset 12–24 hrs. Should not be used in opiate- naive patients
Methadone	**Tablets**—5, 10, 40 mg **Liquid**—Methadone: 1, 2, 10 mg/mL	Consult Pain Specialist	Long	Long half life that is unpredictable. Accumulates with repeated dosing and maximum effect may not be seen until day 2–5. Consultation with someone experienced with methadone is recommended.

The Wilda Assessment

Words to Describe Pain

Aching	Nagging	Stabbing
Burning	Numb	Tender
Dull	Penetrating	Tiring
Exhausting	Radiating	Throbbing
Gnawing	Sharp	Unbearable
Miserable	Shooting	

Pain Intensity Scale

```
10 ———  worst
           possible
            pain

 9 ———

            very
 8 ———    severe
            pain

 7 ———

            severe
 6 ———     pain

 5 ———

            moderate
 4 ———      pain

 3 ———

            mild
 2 ———     pain

 1 ———

            no
 0 ———     pain
```

LOCATIONS OF PAIN

DURATION OF PAIN
Does it hurt all the time
or does it come and go?

Aggravating and/or Alleviating factors
What makes the pain better?
What makes the pain worse?

Analgesic Ladder

Analgesic Reference Guide

Analgesic Ladder
(Adapted from WHO, 1990)

1. Assess pain severity
2. Begin treatment at proper step of ladder
3. Move up ladder until pain controlled

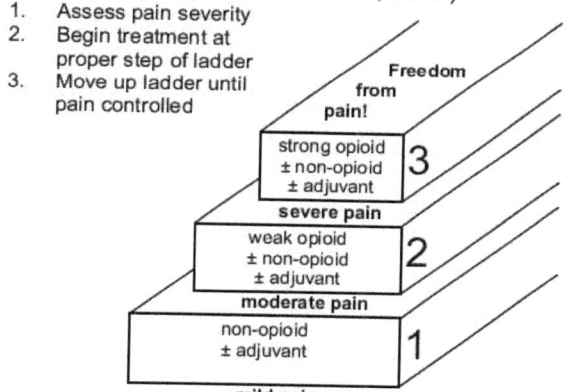

Principles of Pain Management

Principles of Pain Management

1. Use a multi-drug approach by combining opioids with non-opioid adjuvants.

2. Chronic pain almost always requires scheduled and rescue dosing. Scheduled dosing maintains serum levels of medication and provides constant relief. Rescue dosing should be available as needed for breakthrough pain. Frequent rescue dosing indicates a need for increased scheduled medication.

3. Use the dose interval (see Guide inside) for scheduling analgesics. Use long-acting agents for scheduled dosing and short-acting agents for rescue dosing.

4. Use a non-invasive route whenever possible. Acute, severe, or escalating pain may require IV analgesics every 5–15 minutes. If IV dosing must be used for chronic pain, a continuous infusion is indicated.

5. Aggressively manage the side effects of opioids. There is no tolerance to the constipating effects of opioids.

Opioid Conversion Examples

Opioid Conversion Examples
For a patient whose pain is well controlled by 8 Percocet 5 mg/24°: • 8 Percocet is 40 mg Oxydodone/24°, which equals 40 mg MS Contin /24° • Since pain is well controlled, reduce to 30 mg MS Contin /24° (15 mg q12°)   (The dose was reduced by 25% since the pain was well controlled.)

To dose Duragesic patches – total the 24° oral morphine equivalent, divide in half, and apply closest patch size
• For a patient who is taking MS Contin 60 mg q12° and used 4 doses of MSIR 15 mg for breakthrough, 120 + 60 = 180 mg/2 = 90
  – If patient is comfortable use 75 mcg patch
  – If patient's pain is not controlled use 100 mcg patch
• A patient is taking Dilaudid 4 mg PO q 4° (for a total of 24 mg in 24°) the pain is well controlled but need to switch to long-acting opioid for chronic pain.
  – Dilaudid 24mg PO = MS Contin 90 mg/24°
  – pain is controlled (reduce dose by 25%)
  – 90 mg – 22 (25%) = 68, MS Contin 30 mg q 12°, and use Dilaudid 4mg PO q 2° PRN for Breakthrough pain

For a patient who is continuing to feel pain despite Morphine 2 mg/hr IV: • Morphine 2 mg/hr IV = Morphine 48 mg/24° IV = Morphine 144 mg/24° po = Fentanyl 72 mcg TD • The order would read "Duragesic 75 mcg/hr patch q 72°"   (This dose was not reduced since the pain is not yet controlled.)

Adjuvants to Opioid Therapy

Adjuvants to Opioid Therapy	
Adjuvant (Examples)	**Common Indication(s)**
Alpha agonist (clonidine)	neuropathic pain
Anticonvulsants (gabapentin, pregabalin)	neuropathic pain or post-herpetic neuralgia
Antihistamines (diphenhydramine, hydroxyzine, loratadine)	nausea, pruritus, or anxiety
Benzodiazepines (clonazepam, diazepam, lorazepam)	anxiety or myoclonus
Corticosteriods (dexamethasone, prednisone)	nerve compression or anorexia
NSAIDs and COX-2 inhibitors (celecoxib, ibuprofen, naproxen)	musculoskeletal pain
Tricyclic antidepressants (amitriptyline, desipramine, nortriptyline)	neuropathic pain or post-herpetic neuralgia

Medical Guidelines for Specific Diseases

Medical Guidelines
for Specific Diseases

End Stage Dementia

Patients will be considered to be in terminal stage of dementia
if the following criteria are met:

I. Functional Assessment Staging

   A. Even severely demented patients may have a prognosis of up to
two years. Survival time depends on variables such as the
incidence of co-morbidities and the comprehensiveness of care.

   B. The patient should be at or beyond Stage 7 of the Functional
Assessment Staging Scale. (See Appendix)

   C. The patient should show all of the following characteristics:
      1. Unable to ambulate without assistance
      2. Unable to dress without assistance
      3. Unable to bathe properly
      4. Urinary and fecal incontinence, intermittent or constant
      5. No meaningful verbal communication; stereotypical
phrases only or ability to speak is limited to six or fewer
intelligible words.

II. Presence of Medical Complications

   A. The presence of medical co-morbid conditions of sufficient
severity to warrant medical treatment, documented within the
past year, decrease survival in advanced dementia.

   B. Co-morbid Conditions associated with dementia:
      1. Aspiration pneumonia
      2. Pyelonephritis or other upper urinary tract infection
      3. Septicemia
      4. Decubitus ulcers, multiple, stage 3-4
      5. Fever, recurrent after antibiotics

   C. Difficulty swallowing food or refusal to eat, sufficiently severe
that patient cannot maintain sufficient fluid and calorie intake to
sustain life, with patient or surrogate refusing tube feedings or
parenteral nutrition.
      1. Patients who are receiving tube feedings must have
documented impaired nutritional status as indicated by:
         a. Unintentional progressive weight loss >10% over
the prior six months
         b. Serum Albumin <2.5 gm/dl may be a helpful
prognostic indicator, but should not be used by itself

**Considerations: If the patient does not meet the above referenced
guidelines, they may still qualify; consider the present underlying
illness(es)/co-morbidities that may affect the terminality of the
patient's condition.**

National Hospice Organization Copyright 1996

Medical Guidelines for Determining Prognosis in Selected Non-Cancer Diseases, 2nd ed.

End Stage Heart Disease

I. Symptoms of recurrent congestive heart failure (CHF) at rest.

    A. These patients are classified as New York Heart Association (NYHA) Class IV. (See Appendix)

    B. Ejection Fraction of 20% or less is helpful supplemental objective evidence, but should not be required if not already available.

II. Patients should already be optimally treated with diuretics and vasodilators, preferably angiotensin-converting enzyme (ACE) inhibitors.

    A. The patient experiences persistent symptoms of congestive heart failure despite attempts at maximal medical management with diuretics and vasodilators.

    B. "Optimally treated" means that patients who are not on vasodilators have a medical reason for refusing these drugs, e.g. hypotension or renal disease.

    C. Although newer beta blockers with vasodilator activity, e.g. carvedilol, have recently been shown to decrease morbidity and mortality in chronic CHF, they are not included in the definition of "optimal treatment" at this time.

III. In patients with refractory, optimally treated CHF as defined above, each of the following factors have been shown to decrease survival further, and thus may help in educating medical personnel as to the appropriateness of hospice for cardiac patients.

    A. Symptomatic supraventricular or ventricular arrhythmias that are resistant to antiarrhythmic therapy.

    B. History of cardiac arrest and resuscitation in any setting.

    C. History of unexplained syncope.

    D. Cardiogenic brain embolism, i.e., embolic CVA of cardiac origin.

    E. Concomitant HIV disease.

Considerations: If the patient does not meet the above referenced guidelines, they may still qualify; consider the present underlying illness(es)/co-morbidities that may affect the terminality of the patient's condition.

National Hospice Organization Copyright 1996
Medical Guidelines for Determining Prognosis in Selected Non-Cancer Diseases, 2nd ed.

End Stage HIV Disease

I. CD4 + Count
   A. Patients whose CD4+ count is below 25 cells/mcL, measured during a period; when patient is relatively free of acute illness may have a prognosis less than six months, but should be followed clinically and observed for disease progression and decline in recent functional status.
   B. Patients with CD4+ count above 50 cells/mcL, may have a longer prognosis unless there is a non-HIV related co-exisiting life threatening disease.

II. Viral Load
   A. Patients with a persistent HIV RNA (viral load) of >100,000 copies/ml may have a prognosis less than six months.
   B. Patients with lower viral loads may have a prognosis of less than six months if:
      1. They have elected to forego antiretroviral and prophylactic medication
      2. Their functional status is declining
      3. They are experiencing complications listed in III below

III. The following factors have been shown to decrease survival significantly and should be documented if present:
   A. Chronic persistent diarrhea for one year, regardless of etiology
   B. Persistent serum albumin <2.5 gm/dl
   C. Concomitant substance abuse
   D. Age >50
   E. Decisions to forego antiretroviral, chemotherapeutic and prophylactic drug therapy related specifically to HIV disease
   F. Congestive heart failure, symptomatic at rest

Considerations: If the patient does not meet the above referenced guidelines, they may still qualify; consider the present underlying illness(es)/co-morbidities that may affect the terminality of the patient's condition.

End Stage Liver Disease

I. **Laboratory indicators of severely impaired liver function**
The patient should show the following:
   A. Prothrombin time prolonged more than 5 seconds over control
   B. Serum albumin < 2.5gm/dl

II. **Clinical Indicators of end stage liver disease:**
   A. End stage liver disease is present and patient shows at least one of the following:
      1. Ascites, refractory to sodium restriction and diuretics, or patient non-compliant
      2. Spontaneous bacterial peritonitis
      3. Hepatorenal syndrome (elevated creatinine and BUN with oliguria (<400 ml/day) and urine sodium concentration <10 mEq/l
      4. Hepatic encephalopathy, refractory to protein restriction and lactulose or neomycin, or patient non-compliant
      5. Recurrent variceal bleeding, despite intensive therapy

III. **The following factors have been shown to worsen prognosis and should be documented if present.**
      1. Progressive malnutrition
      2. Muscle wasting with reduced strength and endurance
      3. Continued active alcoholism (>80 gm ethanol/day)
      4. Hepatocellular carcinoma
      5. HBsAg (Hepatitis B) positive

Considerations: If the patient does not meet the above referenced guidelines, they may still qualify; consider the present underlying illness(es)/co-morbidities that may affect the terminality of the patient's condition.

National Hospice Organization Copyright 1996
Medical Guidelines for Determining Prognosis in Selected Non-Cancer Diseases, 2nd ed.

End Stage Pulmonary Disease

I. Severity of chronic lung disease documented by:
A. Disabling dyspnea at rest, poorly or unresponsive to bronchodilators, resulting in decreased functional activity, e.g., bed-to-chair existence, often exacerbated by other debilitating symptoms such as fatigue and cough.
Forced Expiratory Volume in One Second (FEV1), after bronchodilator, less than 30% of predicted, is helpful supplemental objective evidence, but should not be required if not already available.
B. Progressive pulmonary disease
  1. Increasing visits to Emergency Department or hospitalizations for pulmonary infections and /or respiratory failure.
  2. Decrease in FEV1 on serial testing of greater than 40 ml per year is helpful supplemental objective evidence, but should not be required if not already available.

II. Presence of cor pulmonale or right heart failure (RHF).
A. These should be due to advanced pulmonary disease, not primary or secondary to left heart disease or valvulopathy.
B. Cor pulmonale may be documented by:
  1. Echocardiography
  2. Electrocardiogram
  3. Chest x-ray
  4. Physical signs of RHF

III. Hypoxemia at rest on supplemental oxygen.
A. $pO2 \leq$ to 55mm Hg on supplemental oxygen.
B. Oxygen saturation $\leq$ or equal to 88% on supplemental oxygen.

IV. Hypercapnia.
A. $pCO2$ equal to or greater than 50mm Hg.

V. Unintentional progressive weight loss >10% of body weight over the preceding six months.

VI. Resting tachycardia > 100/min in a patient with known severe COPD.

Considerations: If the patient does not meet the above referenced guidelines, they may still qualify; consider the present underlying illness(es)/co-morbidities that may affect the terminality of the patient's condition.

National Hospice Organization Copyright 1996
Medical Guidelines for Determining Prognosis in Selected Non-Cancer Diseases, 2nd ed.

End Stage Renal Disease

I. Laboratory criteria for renal failure.

These values may be used to assess patients with renal
failure who are not dialyzed, as well as those who survive
more than a week or two after dialysis is discontinued.

  A. Creatinine clearance of <10cc/min (<15 cc/min for diabetics) AND

  B. Serum creatinine >8.0 mg/dl (>6.0 mg/dl for diabetics).

II. Clinical signs and syndromes associated with renal failure.

  A. Uremia; clinical manifestations of renal failure.

     1. Confusion, obtundation

     2. Intractable nausea and vomiting

     3. Generalized pruritis

     4. Restlessness, "restless legs"

  B. Oliguria: Urine output less than 400cc/24hrs.

  C. Intractable hyperkalemia: persistent serum potassium >7.0 not
responsive to medical management

  D. Uremic pericarditis

  E. Hepatorenal syndrome

  F. Intractable fluid overload

**III. Acute Renal Failure: co-morbid conditions may predict
early mortality:**

     1. Mechanical Ventilation

     2. Malignancy – other organ systems

     3. Chronic lung disease

     4. Advanced Cardiac or Liver Disease

     5. Sepsis

     6. Immunosupression/AIDS

     7. Albumin <3.5gm/dl

     8. Cachexia

     9. Platelet count <25,000

     10. Age >75

     11. Disseminated intravascular coagulation

     12. Gastrointestinal bleeding

**Considerations: If the patient does not meet the above referenced
guidelines, they may still qualify; consider the present underlying
illness(es)/co-morbidities that may affect the terminality of the
patient's condition.**

End Stage Stroke and Coma

I. During the acute phase immediately following a hemorrhagic or ischemic stroke, any of the following are strong predictors of early mortality:

   A. Coma or persistent vegetative state secondary to stroke, beyond three day's duration.

   B. In post-anoxic stroke, coma or severe obtundation, accompanied by severe myoclonus, persisting beyond three days past the anoxic event.

   C. Comatose patients with any 4 of the following on day 3 of coma had 97% mortality by two months:

      1. Abnormal brain stem response
      2. Absent verbal response
      3. Absent withdrawal response to pain
      4. Serum creatinine >1.5mg/dl
      5. Age>70

   D. Dysphagia severe enough to prevent the patient from receiving food and fluids necessary to sustain life, in a patient who declines, or is not a candidate for, artificial nutrition and hydration.

   E. If computed tomographic (CT) or magnetic resonance imaging (MRI) scans are available, certain specific findings may indicate decreased likelihood of survival, or at least poor prognosis for recovery of function even with vigorous rehabilitation efforts, which may influence decisions concerning life support or hospice.

II. Chronic Phase, the following clinical factors may correlate with poor survival in the setting of severe stroke, and should be documented.

   A. Age >70

   B. Poor functional status, as evidenced by Karnofsky score of <50%.

   C. Post-stroke dementia, as evidenced by a FAST score of greater than 7.

   D. Poor nutritional status, whether on artificial nutrition or not:

      1. Unintentional progressive weight loss of greater than 10% over past six months
      2. Serum albumin less than 2.5 gm/dl may be a helpful prognostic indicator, but should not be used by itself

   E. Medical complications related to debility and progressive clinical decline:

      1. Aspiration pneumonia
      2. Upper urinary tract infection
      3. Sepsis
      4. Refractory stage 3-4 decubitus ulcers
      5. Fever recurrent after antibiotics

Considerations: If the patient does not meet the above referenced guidelines, they may still qualify; consider the present underlying illness(es)/co-morbidities that may affect the terminality of the patient's condition.

National Hospice Organization Copyright 1996
Medical Guidelines for Determining Prognosis in Selected Non-Cancer Diseases, 2nd ed.

General Debility

I. The patient's condition is life-limiting, and the patient and/or family have been informed of this determination.

      1. A "life-limiting condition" may be due to a specific diagnosis, a combination of diseases, or there may be no specific diagnosis defined.

II. The patient and/or family have elected treatment goals directed toward relief of symptoms, rather than cure of the underlying disease.

III. The patient has either of the following:

  A. Documented clinical progression of disease, which may include:

      1. Progression of the primary disease process as listed in disease-specific criteria, as documented by physician assessment, laboratory, radiologic or other studies

      2. Multiple Emergency Department visits or inpatient hospitalizations over the prior six months

      3. For homebound patients receiving home health services, nursing assessment may be documented

      4. A recent decline in functional status may be documented

         a. Diminished functional status may be documented by either:

            1. Karnofsky Performance Status of less than or equal to 50% or

            2. Dependence in at least three of six ADL's

               a. Bathing

               b. Dressing

               c. Feeding

               d. Transfers

               e. Continence of bowel and bladder

               f. Ability to ambulate independently to BR

  B. Documented recent impaired nutritional status related to the terminal process:

      1. Unintentional, progressive weight loss of greater than 10% over the prior six months

      2. Serum albumin less than 2.5gm/dl may be a helpful prognostic indicator, but should not be used in isolation

Amyotrophic Lateral Sclerosis (ALS)

I. **Rapid progression of disease and critically impaired ventilatory capacity.**

   A. Rapid progression of ALS. Most of the disability should have developed in past 12 months.

      1. Progressing from independent ambulation to wheelchair or bed-bound status

      2. Progressing from normal to barely intelligible or unintelligible speech

      3. Progressing from normal to pureed diet

      4. Progressing from independence in most or all ADL's to requiring assistance in all ADL's.

   B. Critically impaired ventilatory capacity.

      1. Vital capacity (VC) less than 30% of predicted

      2. Significant dyspnea at rest

      3. Requiring supplement oxygen at rest

      4. Patient declines artificial ventilation

II. **Rapid progression of ALS and critical nutritional impairment.**

      1. Oral intake or nutrients and fluids insufficient to sustain life.

      2. Continued weight loss

      3. Dehydration or hypovolemia

      4. Absence of artificial feeding methods

III. **Rapid progression of ALS and life-threatening complications.**

      1. Recurrent aspiration pneumonia (with or without tube feedings)

      2. Decubitus ulcers, multiple, Stage 3-4, particularly if infected

      3. Upper urinary tract infections, e.g. pyelonephritis

      4. Sepsis

      5. Recurrent fever after antibiotic therapy

Considerations: If the patient does not meet the above referenced guidelines, they may still qualify; consider the present underlying illness(es)/co-morbidities that may affect the terminality of the patient's condition.

National Hospice Organization Copyright 1996
Medical Guidelines for Determining Prognosis in Selected Non-Cancer Diseases, 2nd ed.

Functional Assessment Staging (FAST Scale)

Functional Assessment Staging (Fast)

(Check highest consecutive level of disability)

1. No difficulty either subjectively or objectively.
2. Complains of forgetting location of objects. Subjective work difficulties.
3. Decreased job functioning evident to co-workers. Difficulty in traveling to new locations. Decreased organizational capacity.*
4. Decreased ability to perform complex tasks, e.g. planning dinner for guests, handling personal finances (such as forgetting to pay bills), difficulty marketing, etc.
5. Requires assistance in choosing proper clothing to wear for the day, season or occasion, e.g. patient may wear the same clothing repeatedly, unless supervised.*
6. A) Improperly putting on clothes without assistance or prompting (e.g. may put street clothes on over night clothes, or put shoes on wrong feet, or have difficulty buttoning clothing) occasionally or more frequently over the past weeks.*

    B) Unable to bathe properly (e.g., difficulty adjusting bath-water temp.) occasionally or more frequently over the past weeks.*

    C) Inability to handle mechanics of toileting (e.g., forgets to flush the toilet, does not wipe properly or properly dispose of toilet tissue) occasionally or more frequently over the past weeks.*

    D) Urinary incontinence (occasionally or more frequently over the past weeks).*

    E) Fecal incontinence (occasionally or more frequently over the past weeks).*

7. A) Ability to speak limited to approximately a half dozen intelligible different words or fewer, in the course of an average day or in the course of an intensive interview.

    B) Speech ability is limited to the use of a single intelligible word in an average day or in the course of an intensive interview (the person may repeat the word over and over).

    C) Ambulatory ability is lost (cannot walk without personal assistance).

    D) Cannot sit up without assistance (e.g., the individual will fall over if there are not lateral rests [arms] on the chair).

    E) Loss of ability to smile.

    F) Loss of ability to hold up head independently.

*Scored primarily on the basis of information obtained from acknowledgeable informant and/or category.

National Hospice Organization Copyright 1996
Medical Guidelines for Determining Prognosis in Selected Non-Cancer Diseases, 2nd ed.

Palliative Performance Scale (PPS)

%	Ambulation	Activity and Evidence of Disease	Self-Care	Intake	Conscious Level
100	Full	Normal activity No evidence of disease	Full	Normal	Full
90	Full	Normal activity Some evidence of disease	Full	Normal	Full
80	Full	Normal activity with effort Some evidence of disease	Full	Normal or reduced	Full
70	Reduced	Unable to do normal job/work Some evidence of disease	Full	Normal or reduced	Full
60	Reduced	Unable to do hobby/house work Significant disease	Occasional Assistance Necessary	Normal or reduced	Full or confusion
50	Mainly sit/lie	Unable to do any work Extensive disease	Considerable Assistance Required	Normal or reduced	Full or confusion
40	Mainly in bed	As above	Mainly assistance	Normal or reduced	Full or drowsy or confusion
30	Totally bed-bound	As above	Total care	Reduced	Full or drowsy or confusion
20	As above	As above	Total care	Minimal to sips	Full or drowsy or confusion
10	As above	As above	Total care	Mouth care only	Drowsy or coma
0	Death	---	---	---	---

1. To determine the PPS Score, begin at the left column ("Ambulation") and read down until the "best fit" is found. Circle it.
2. Then look at the next column to the right, "Activity and Evidence of Disease," and read down again until the best fit is found. Circle it.
3. Continue evaluating the best fit for all five steps.
4. Then determine the Best Fit Score.
5. PPS scores are only in 10% increments (there is no such score as 42% or 35%).

Anderson F, et al. Palliative Performance Scale (PPS): A New Tool. J Palliative Care 1996; 12(1): 5–11.

Weight Chart for Women

Weight in pounds, based on ages 25-59 with the lowest mortality rate
(indoor clothing weighing 3 pounds and shoes with 1" heels)

Height	Small Frame	Medium Frame	Large Frame
4'10"	102-111	109-121	118-131
4'11"	103-113	111-123	120-134
5'0"	104-115	113-126	122-137
5'1"	106-118	115-129	125-140
5'2"	108-121	118-132	128-143
5'3"	111-124	121-135	131-147
5'4"	114-127	124-138	134-151
5'5"	117-130	127-141	137-155
5'6"	120-133	130-144	140-159
5'7"	123-136	133-147	143-163
5'8"	126-139	136-150	146-167
5'9"	129-142	139-153	149-170
5'10"	132-145	142-156	152-173
5'11"	135-148	145-159	155-176
6'0"	138-151	148-162	158-179

http://healthchecksystems.com/heightweightchart.htm

Weight Chart for Men

Weight in pounds, based on ages 25-59 with the lowest mortality rate
(indoor clothing weighing 5 pounds and shoes with 1" heels)

Height	Small Frame	Medium Frame	Large Frame
5'2"	128-134	131-141	138-150
5'3"	130-136	133-143	140-153
5'4"	132-138	135-145	142-156
5'5"	134-140	137-148	144-160
5'6"	136-142	139-151	146-164
5'7"	138-145	142-154	149-168
5'8"	140-148	145-157	152-172
5'9"	142-151	148-160	155-176
5'10"	144-154	151-163	158-180
5'11"	146-157	154-166	161-184
6'0"	149-160	157-170	164-188
6'1"	152-164	160-174	168-192
6'2"	155-168	164-178	172-197
6'3"	158-172	167-182	176-202
6'4"	162-176	171-187	181-207

http://healthchecksystems.com/heightweightchart.htm

Calculating Your Frame Size

Following is the method the Metropolitan Life Insurance Company used to calculate frame size:

1. Extend your arm in front of your body bending your elbow at a ninety degree angle to your body so that your forearm is parallel to your body.

2. Keep your fingers straight and turn the inside of your wrist towards your body.

3. Place your thumb and index finger on the two prominent bones on either side of your elbow, then measure the distance between the bones with a tape measure or calipers.

4. Compare to the chart below. The chart lists elbow measurements for a medium frame - if your elbow measurement for that particular height is less than the number of inches listed, you are a small frame - if your elbow measurement for that particular height is more than the number of inches listed, you are a large frame.

Elbow Measurements for Medium Frame

Men	Elbow Measurement	Women	Elbow Measurement
5'2" - 5'3"	2-1/2" to 2-7/8"	4'10"-4'11"	2-1/4" to 2-1/2"
5'4" - 5'7"	2-5/8" to 2-7/8"	5'0" - 5'3"	2-1/4" to 2-1/2"
5'8" - 5'11"	2-3/4" to 3"	5'4" - 5'7"	2-3/8" to 2-5/8"
6'0" - 6'3"	2-3/4" to 3-1/8"	5'8" - 5'11"	2-3/8" to 2-5/8"
6'4"	2-7/8" to 3-1/4"	6'0"	2-1/2" to 2-3/4"

Weight Table for Women Aged 65 and Older

Height In Inches	Age 65-69	Age 70-74	Age 75-79	Age 80-84	Age 85-89	Age 90-94
58	120-146	112-138	111-135	--	--	--
59	121-147	114-140	112-136	100-122	99-121	--
60	122-148	118-142	113-139	108-130	102-124	--
61	123-151	118-144	115-141	109-133	104-128	--
62	125-153	121-147	118-144	112-138	108-132	107-131
63	127-155	123-151	121-147	115-141	112-136	107-131
64	130-158	128-154	123-151	119-145	115-141	108-132
65	132-162	130-158	126-154	122-150	120-146	112-136
66	136-166	132-162	128-157	126-154	124-152	116-142
67	140-170	136-166	131-161	130-158	128-156	--
68	143-175	140-170	--	--	--	--
69	148-180	144-176				

Adapted from Journal of the American Medical Association, Vol. 177, p. 558, with permission of American Medical Association. Copyright 1980, American Medical Association.

Weight Table for Men Aged 65 and Older

Height In Inches	Age 65-69	Age 70-74	Age 75-79	Age 80-84	Age 85-89	Age 90-94
61	128-158	125-153	123-151	--	--	--
62	130-158	127-155	125-153	122-148	--	--
63	131-151	129-157	127-155	122-150	120-146	--
64	134-154	131-161	129-157	124-152	122-148	--
65	136-166	134-164	130-160	127-155	125-153	117-143
66	138-169	137-167	133-163	130-158	128-156	120-148
67	140-172	140-170	136-166	132-162	130-160	122-150
68	143-175	142-174	139-169	135-165	133-163	126-154
69	147-179	146-178	142-174	139-169	137-167	130-158
70	150-184	148-182	146-178	143-175	140-172	134-164
71	155-189	152-186	149-183	148-180	144-176	139-169
72	159-195	156-190	154-188	153-187	148-182	--
73	164-200	160-196	158-192	--	--	--

Adapted from Journal of the American Medical Association, Vol. 177, p. 558, with permission of American Medical Association. Copyright 1980, American Medical Association.

Stages of Heart Disease

NYHA Classification

In order to determine the best course of therapy, physicians often assess the stages of heart failure according to the New York Heart Associations (NYHA) functional classification system. This system relates symptoms everyday activities and the patient's quality of life.

Class	Patient Symptoms
Class I (Mild)	No Limitation of physical activity, ordinary physical activity does not cause undue fatigue, palpitation, or dyspnea (shortness of breath).
Class II (Mild)	Slight limitation of physical activity, comfortable at rest, but ordinary physical activity results in fatigue, palpitation, or dyspnea.
Class III (Moderate)	Marked limitation of physical activity comfortable at rest, but less than ordinary activity causes fatigue, palpitation, or dyspnea.
Class IV (Severe)	Unable to carry out any physical activity without discomfort. Symptoms of cardiac insufficiency at rest. If any physical activity is undertaken, discomfort is increased.

National Hospice Organization Copyright 1996
Medical Guidelines for Determining Prognosis in Selected Non-Cancer Diseases, 2nd ed.

Index

Page numbers in *italics* denote figures; those followed by a t denote tables.

Debility, 102–103
    documenting, 281–282t
Decisional/decision-making ability,
        57–58
    criteria for, 57
    decisional thresholds, 58
    defined, 57
    pitfalls, 58
    time specific, 58
Dehydration, benefits of when dying, 155
Delirium, 159–161
    agitated/hyperactive, 127
    defined, 124
    dementia *vs.*, 128, 160
    in dying patients, 135
    features of, 159–160
    hypoactive-hypoalert, 127
    management of, 160
    near death awareness *vs.*, 124
    origin of, 160
    psychomotor abnormalities and, 159
    sleep/wake cycle abnormalities and,
        159
    terminal, 127–129
    treatment of opioid-induced, 200t
Dementia
    delirium *vs.*, 128, 160
    end-stage, 282–283t
    prognosis for, 99
    tube feeding and advanced, 237
Depression, 166
    decisional ability and, 58
Desipramine, for pain, 184
Desitin ointment, 165
Dexamethasone
    for pain, 184
    for pruritus, 169
Dextroamphetamine, for sedation side
        effect, 200t
Diaphragm, irritation of, 151
Diarrhea, 162–163
    diet for, 163
    evaluation of, 162
    reintroducing solids, 163
    skin problems and, 163
    treatment of, 162–163
Diazepam
    methadone and, 214
    for pain, 184

Dickinson, Emily, 5
Diet, for diarrhea, 163
Digoxin, delirium and, 160
Diphenhydramine (Benadryl)
    for insomnia, 171
    for pain, 184
    for pruritus, 169, 200t, 206
Diphenoxylate/atropine (Lomotil), for
        diarrhea, 162
Disease, chronic, 10–11
Ditropan (oxybutrynin), for inconti-
        nence, 164
Diuretics, 138
Diverting ostomy, 250
Dizziness, 149–150
    teaching for caregivers, 149–150
    treatment of, 149
DNR. *See* Do Not Resuscitate
Documentation
    of action, 287
    comparing to "normal" person, 280
    of death, 73–74
    of debility/failure to thrive, 281–282t
    of end-stage cardiac disease, 283t
    of end-stage dementia, 282–283t
    of end-stage liver disease, 285t
    of end-stage neurologic disease and
            cerebrovascular accident,
            286–287t
    of end-stage pulmonary disease,
            284–285t
    of end-stage renal disease, 283–284t
    of family meeting, 37
    interdisciplinary care and, 287
    language used in, 281
    mnemonics, 280t
    negative, 279–280
    in palliative care, 279–287
    of ventilator withdrawal, 246
Domeboro soaks, 170
Do Not Resuscitate (DNR) orders,
        51–53
    African Americans and use of, 18
    clarifying future plans and, 53
    discussing, 52
    patient understanding of, 52
    in seriously ill patients, 53
Dose escalation, for pain control, 184
DPOA. *See* Durable power of attorney